The Good CPD Guide

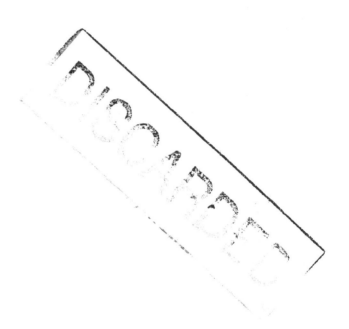

The Good CPD Guide

A practical guide to managed continuing
professional development in medicine

Second Edition

Janet Grant
Professor of Education in Medicine
Centre for Education in Medicine
The Open University

Foreword by
Thomas Zilling
Associate Professor of Surgery, Lund University, Sweden
President, Swedish Association of Senior Hospital Physicians
Vice President, European Association of Senior Hospital Physicians

Radcliffe Publishing
London • New York

Radcliffe Publishing Ltd
33–41 Dallington Street
London
EC1V 0BB
United Kingdom

www.radcliffepublishing.com

Electronic catalogue and worldwide online ordering facility.

British Library Cataloguing in Publication Data.

A catalogue record for this book is available from the British Library.

ISBN-13: 978 184619 570 9

The paper used for the text pages of this book is FSC® certified. FSC (The Forest Stewardship Council®) is an international network to promote responsible management of the world's forests.

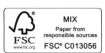

Typeset by Phoenix Photosetting, Chatham, Kent
Printed and bound by TJI Digital, Padstow, Cornwall

Contents

Foreword

CPD FOR CHANGE

Continuing professional development is unquestioned in modern-day society. Knowledge-intensive organisations have to invest in their employees in order to survive. This is especially important for the medical profession. Once specialist certification has been achieved, the continuing process of lifelong learning is in many countries unspecified. Cutbacks in funding for healthcare and a shortage of doctors have brought into focus medical productivity and given ongoing development and training of staff a lower priority. At the same time, one of the most important challenges for doctors today is to raise the competencies needed to increase patient safety and improve healthcare. With this in mind, we are entering a political arena where CPD, in its limited form sometimes still called Continuing Medical Education (CME), is used by some governments and authorities to regulate mandatory learning standards for doctors. Today there is a diversity of CPD systems worldwide, ranging from entirely voluntary to mandatory by law. These are usually based on collecting credit points, as an indicator of CPD activity. In some countries mandatory systems involve a revalidation or recertification process run by either government authorities or professional bodies.

A structure and process for CPD is necessary but not always at hand. Thus, the new expanded second edition of *The Good CPD Guide* by Professor Janet Grant is such an important contribution and fills the much needed gap, especially since this comprehensive guide is based on evidence from current literature studies, along with practical experience from the United Kingdom.

The Good CPD Guide includes all aspects of CPD such as *quality improvement* – the actual process of CPD or managed CPD – *quality assurance* – a system for physicians to prove to the public that they are capable of delivering top-notch healthcare – and, finally, *quality control* – in the meaning of recertification as applied in some countries.

The Good CPD Guide gives examples of how to introduce and follow up CPD, and challenges countries with mandatory CPD systems based only on CME-credit points to broaden and enhance their offerings. Professor Grant's recommendations advocate integrated learning, uniting theory and practice, in an educationally friendly environment.

The development of CPD in the USA can also serve as an example for change where systems for recertification and revalidation were introduced during the seventies. The Americans have gradually changed from CME towards CPD. A good example is the 'General Competencies' from The Accreditation Council for Graduate Medical Education (www.acgme.org) which include: 1 Patient care, 2 Medical knowledge, 3 Practice-based learning and improvement, 4 Interpersonal and communication skills, 5 Professionalism, and 6 Systems-based practice. Professor Grant's CPD guide goes deeper and beyond these areas.

CPD is the key to excellent healthcare. Professional ethics should drive the system and there should be adequate resources for the development of the structure and process of CPD. This second edition of *The Good CPD Guide* is the roadmap to where we stand today and where we are heading. This guide will inspire not only physicians but also administrators, government officials and healthcare organisations. This book is a must for everyone engaged in CPD for the medical profession.

Dr Thomas Zilling MD, PhD
Associate Professor of Surgery, Lund University, Sweden
President, Swedish Association of Senior Hospital Physicians
Vice President, European Association of Senior Hospital Physicians
September 2011

About the author

Janet is an educational psychologist and Professor of Education in Medicine at the UK Open University Centre for Education in Medicine (OUCEM). Her special interest is in how students, trainees and experienced doctors develop knowledge and skill, and on the relationship between medical education and clinical practice.

Janet works both nationally and internationally on medical education development and regulation. She is an honorary member of three medical Royal Colleges.

Acknowledgements

This new edition of *The Good CPD Guide* owes a lot to the work of those who developed the first edition (1999). Subsequent research and policy development have shown that the guidance and the conclusions of that edition remain unchanged, even though the details of context have altered.

We would, therefore, like to acknowledge the work of the following key players:

Ellie Chambers

Dr Gordon Jackson

Mr Robert Atlay

Dr Peter Bourdillon

Dr Claire du Boulay

Dr Shelley Heard

Dr Mike Isaac

Dr Doug Justins

Dr Gay Kingsley

Dr Peter Luce

Mr Peter Milton

Mr Vincent O'Neill

Prof Trudie Roberts

Dr Frank Smith

Mr Adrian Steger

Mr Paul Thomas

Dr Alistair Thomson

Dr Peter Toghill

Mr Denis Wilkins

Dr Helen Mulholland

Introduction: What is managed continuing professional development?

BACKGROUND

The role of continuing professional development (CPD) is now centre-stage in the minds of regulators, educationalists and the profession. In terms of continued fitness to practise and patient safety, as well as maintaining professional standards, a more thoughtful and transparent approach to CPD has gradually become the accepted aim.

There are many competing and complementary definitions of CPD, depending on the main perspective; thus, for example, CPD can be:

> 'A continuing process, outside formal undergraduate and postgraduate training, that allows individual doctors to maintain and improve standards of medical practice through the development of knowledge, skills, attitudes and behaviour. CPD should also support specific changes in practice.'[1]

Or it is:

> '... a continuing learning process that complements formal undergraduate and postgraduate education and training. CPD requires doctors to maintain and improve their standards across all areas of their practice ... CPD should also encourage and support specific changes in practice and career development.'[2]

There is some debate about exactly how CPD can be mindful of its various imperatives.

➤ How can CPD be transparent and accountable?
➤ How can CPD be regulated?
➤ How can CPD be relevant to the needs of a developing healthcare service?
➤ How can CPD be relevant to the needs of the individual clinician?
➤ How can CPD be cost effective?
➤ How can a CPD system ensure that the method of learning is effective?

The Good CPD Guide attempts to answer these pressing questions. We will do so by presenting:

➤ An overview of CPD practice
➤ An overview of CPD policy
➤ An analysis of the evidence about the effectiveness of CPD.

Presentation of a system of managed CPD that answers the questions put above.

We also present management tools and documentation for CPD, as well as describing ways of identifying learning needs, undertaking related learning and reinforcing that learning.

WHAT IS MANAGED CPD?

Managed CPD is a systematic approach to continuing learning and development for medical practitioners which will:

➤ Relate CPD to the needs of the changing and developing healthcare service

➤ Ensure the personal and professional development of the individual doctor

➤ Provide an accountable and transparent system which can be used for regulatory, quality assurance, revalidation and relicensure purposes.

The approach to managed CPD presented is based on the published literature, the professional and regulatory environment, and on the established practice of doctors who have integrated their own continuing learning and development with the provision of patient care. We have no reason to believe other than that the vast majority of doctors are already lifelong learners who take their own current knowledge and skill very seriously indeed.

It is those good doctors to whom we turned to determine how they do, actually, keep themselves up to date.

The Good CPD managed process can be seen as the stages of What? How? Learn Use:

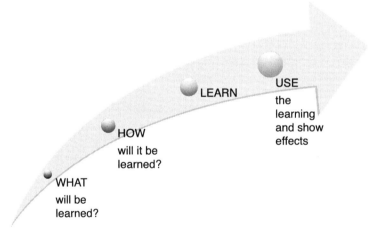

Figure 1: The Good CPD managed process

This process of managed CPD is described further in Figure 2. The process outlined is based on the:

➤ published literature on the effectiveness of CPD
➤ need for CPD to be incorporated into the regulatory process
➤ actual approaches of doctors in keeping themselves up to date.

Managed CPD not only responds to the demands of the regulatory system, but also recognises that doctors have different learning needs, learn in different ways and in different contexts.

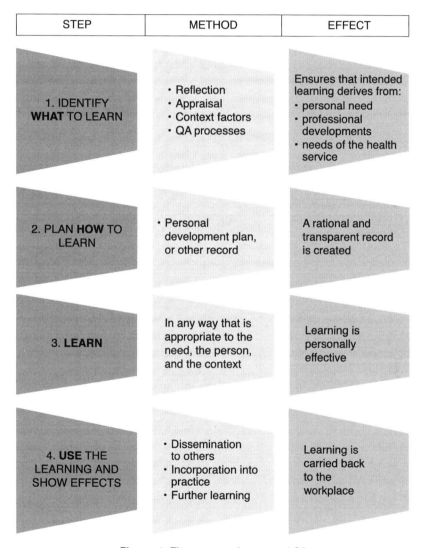

STEP	METHOD	EFFECT
1. IDENTIFY **WHAT** TO LEARN	• Reflection • Appraisal • Context factors • QA processes	Ensures that intended learning derives from: • personal need • professional developments • needs of the health service
2. PLAN **HOW** TO LEARN	• Personal development plan, or other record	A rational and transparent record is created
3. **LEARN**	In any way that is appropriate to the need, the person, and the context	Learning is personally effective
4. **USE** THE LEARNING AND SHOW EFFECTS	• Dissemination to others • Incorporation into practice • Further learning	Learning is carried back to the workplace

Figure 2: The system of managed CP

Each of these components is discussed in the following chapters.

HOW DOES MANAGED CPD FIT INTO PROFESSIONAL AND REGULATORY ENVIRONMENTS?

Lord Patel's 2010 report to the UK General Medical Council[3] states that:

> 'Once outside formal training programmes, the onus is on doctors to demonstrate that they are maintaining appropriate professional standards. The role of the regulator is to support them in doing this and to monitor that it is done.
>
> Good Medical Practice requires doctors to keep their knowledge and skills up to date and encourages them to "take part in educational activities that maintain and further develop" their competence and performance. In future, revalidation will provide a focus for that formative activity. These elements will be brought together through appraisal and continuing professional development (CPD) and through each doctor's Personal Development Plan.'

This picture is rapidly becoming the norm in a number of countries. CPD is closely involved in professional development, service development, self-regulation and external regulation. As such, it must be a transparent process that is amenable to record. Some believe that the increasing regulatory burden of revalidation will bring about positive changes in CPD itself.[4] There are many variations in CPD policy between countries in terms of:

➤ Whether CPD is mandatory or not
➤ Which authority regulates CPD
➤ The way in which compliance is counted and monitored (CPD credits which tend to be counted as hours are the most common framework)
➤ The implicit model of learning
➤ What activities are recognised for CPD purposes
➤ Whether CPD providers and events are accredited or formally approved
➤ The consequences of complying or not complying with any CPD targets
➤ Relationship to relicensure or revalidation of registration.

These variations occur because of a relatively poor evidence base, different regulatory régimes, different ownership of the process and different purposes. The design of CPD systems is therefore open to local judgment and context.

Although there are such variations between countries in the way CPD (also still called continuing medical education, or CME, in many countries, including the USA) is conducted, there are some commonly occurring themes.

> The measurement of participation in CPD by accumulation of credits, or hours, is perhaps the most commonly applied framework. Evidence would suggest that it is probably not effective in ensuring that CPD has an impact on practice. Managed CPD addresses this issue.

Common themes, internationally, relate to regulation of the profession, relicensure of the individual doctor, quality assurance, and accreditation of CPD events, as well as the specification of recognised learning methods that will accrue CPD credits. Found within these broad headings are a number of specific entities such as portfolios, appraisal, and other forms of recorded activity. These themes and entities are presented in Figure 4, in relation to the ability of a managed CPD system to cope.

The process of managed CPD described here takes advantage of existing mechanisms within the service and the profession: audit, critical incident methods, peer review, appraisal and other quality assurance measures can not only contribute to needs assessment[5], but also to learning itself, and reinforcement of that learning. Current proposals for appraisal to be at the heart of revalidation[6] ensure harmony between managed CPD and professional relicensing. In this context, four influences on continuing medical education (as the authors term it) have been identified[7], as follows (Figure 3), which managed CPD likewise takes into account:

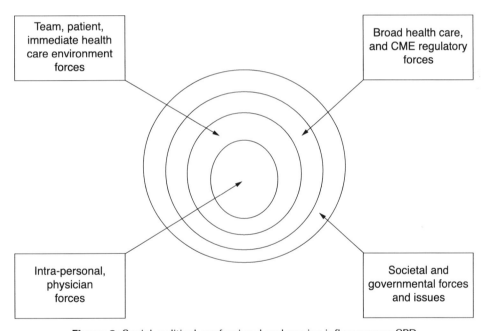

Figure 3: Social, political, professional and service influences on CPD

Schostak *et al.*[8] (2010) concluded that:

'... CPD is valued and is seen as effective when it addresses the needs of individual clinicians, the populations they serve and the organisations within which they work.'

Managed CPD does all of these things.

The World Federation for Medical Education has set out global standards for continuing professional development.[9] These recognise the factors identified in Figure 4.

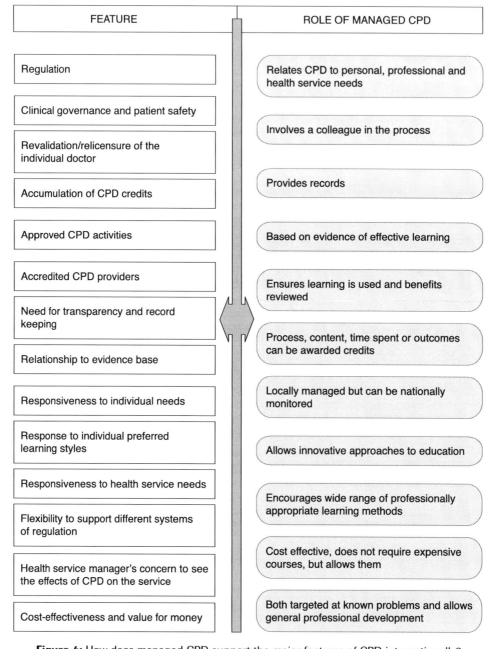

FEATURE	ROLE OF MANAGED CPD
Regulation	Relates CPD to personal, professional and health service needs
Clinical governance and patient safety	Involves a colleague in the process
Revalidation/relicensure of the individual doctor	Provides records
Accumulation of CPD credits	
Approved CPD activities	Based on evidence of effective learning
Accredited CPD providers	Ensures learning is used and benefits reviewed
Need for transparency and record keeping	Process, content, time spent or outcomes can be awarded credits
Relationship to evidence base	Locally managed but can be nationally monitored
Responsiveness to individual needs	
Response to individual preferred learning styles	Allows innovative approaches to education
Responsiveness to health service needs	Encourages wide range of professionally appropriate learning methods
Flexibility to support different systems of regulation	Cost effective, does not require expensive courses, but allows them
Health service manager's concern to see the effects of CPD on the service	Both targeted at known problems and allows general professional development
Cost-effectiveness and value for money	

Figure 4: How does managed CPD support the major features of CPD internationally?

WFME states that:

'Motivation for CPD, from the perspective of the individual doctor, derives from three main sources:

➤ The professional drive to provide optimal care for the individual patient;
➤ The obligation to honour the demands from employers and society;
➤ The need to preserve job satisfaction and prevent "burn out".

The best available evidence suggests that effective CPD is characterised by the presence of four factors:

➤ a clear need or reason for the particular CPD to be undertaken (what will be learned?);
➤ a plan for learning (how will the learning occur?);
➤ learning based on such an identified need or reason (learn);
➤ and follow-up provision for reinforcing the learning accomplished (use).'

Managed CPD shows that CPD credits should be given for a cycle comprising these four steps, rather than for isolated learning events.

MANAGED CPD, CLINICAL GOVERNANCE AND REGULATION

It can be seen from Figure 3 that managed CPD also suits all the necessary conditions of clinical governance which are:

'... a system through which NHS organisations are accountable for continuously improving the quality of their services and safeguarding high standards of care by creating an environment in which excellence in clinical care will flourish.'[10]

The other side of this coin is regulation. Effective regulation, whether driven by the profession itself or by independent or government agencies, must have certain features. The 2005 Hampton review of regulation[11] in the UK applied to business but has since been generalised (whether appropriately or not) to all other regulatory arenas. It suggested some principles:

➤ comprehensive risk assessment should be the foundation of all regulators' enforcement programmes;
➤ there should be no inspections without a reason;
➤ resources released from unnecessary inspections should be redirected towards advice to improve compliance;
➤ there should be fewer, simpler forms;
➤ data requirements, including the design of forms, should be coordinated across regulators;
➤ when new regulations are being devised, departments should plan to ensure that enforcement can be as efficient as possible;
➤ there should be fewer regulators.

Although a risk-based approach to regulation has not, perhaps, been the success that Hampton intended, it is clear that his general approach is one of light-touch on the basis of a sound assessment of likely risks. He advocates guidance, fewer forms, efficiency and a reduced regulatory burden. The approach to CPD designed here, complies with all those imperatives, as the following chart shows:

Hampton principle	Managed CPD compliance
Light-touch	Records are streamlined and easily submitted, if required
Assessment of likely risk	Based on evidence of effective CPD, with peer appraisal to confirm the process
Guidance	The CPD cycle is clearly set out, and is comprehensible because it relates to existing practice, and can be supported by accessible documentation
Fewer forms	Records of the CPD cycle are straightforward
Efficiency	Fits in with existing practice
Reduced regulatory burden	Regulators are not required to introduce new systems or alien processes specifically for regulation

In the UK, regulators of the medical profession take a view about their role in relation to CPD. In a 2010 report commissioned by the General Medical Council (GMC) and the Academy of Medical Royal Colleges, it was observed that:

> 'CPD was often closely associated in the literature with appraisal and revalidation and was also linked to performance...'[12]

In Lord Patel's report 'Recommendations and Options for the Future Regulation of Education and Training'[3] he recommended that the GMC should update its 2004 CPD guidance and re-examine how its regulatory role in CPD should be exercised. This work began in 2010.

Although the GMC had not regulated CPD at that time*, the 2004 GMC guidance indicated their thinking about the relationship between CPD and regulation:

> 'You must keep your knowledge and skills up to date throughout your working life. In particular, you should take part regularly in educational activities which maintain and further develop your competence and performance.'[13]

More recently, it is clear that CPD will play a significant part in the revalidation of the doctor's registration[14] which is a primary regulatory function. Pringle[15] points out that revalidation will involve strengthened annual appraisal, but that:

---

*And at the time of publication still does not do so directly.

'... the main benefit will be in providing regular reassurance that doctors are keeping up to date, reflecting on their care, and developing year on year.'

These purposes are co-terminus with those of managed CPD.

But CPD can have a number of other purposes, as outlined by the Basel Declaration of the UEMS[16]:

i improve the safety and quality of medical practice
ii to encourage lifelong learning
iii to make transparent the outcomes, processes and systems required.

These purposes are not objective, but simply depend, partially, on the agency, whether that is a professional body, a regulator or an educationalist.

Whatever the purpose, however, they have the safety and improvement of a doctor's practice in common. That being the case, we should consider how CPD can be a part of this inevitable developmental process. Achieving a balance between the needs of the clinician and the service has not always been easy.[17]

THE EFFECTIVENESS OF CONTINUING PROFESSIONAL DEVELOPMENT

In 2000, a review of the literature concerning the effectiveness of CPD for the United Kingdom's Chief Medical Officer,[18] found that:

'The key to effectiveness of CPD is not to be found in the learning methods adopted. There is no best learning method or approach to learning. Instead, the key to effectiveness is to make sure the process of CPD is effectively managed to have the following components:

1. A stated reason for the CPD to be undertaken. This might be specific (for example, a need to develop a new skill). Or, it might be a general professional reason (for example, a wish to undertake general professional updating with colleagues at a conference). It might also arise from the needs of the service (for example, to develop a skill that offers new areas of care to patients).
2. An identified method of learning which might be formal or informal
3. Some follow-up after the CPD for reinforcement and dissemination of the learning that can also demonstrate its benefits. This might be actions such as reporting back to colleagues, developing new services, demonstrating new skills, or simply feeling more confident.

These conclusions match those of Davis *et al.*,[19] in their review of randomised controlled trials[20] of CPD.'

The more recent review conducted for the UK Academy of Medical Royal Colleges and the General Medical Council, reaches the same conclusion.[8] Such a conclusion would also support the Swedish Medical Association's four-step guidance[21] which gives the following advice:

1. Analyse the need and start the process
2. Develop supporting functions
3. Collaborate
4. Follow up and evaluate.

In the wake of increasing interest in CPD, our 2000 literature review has been updated for this new edition of *The Good CPD Guide*. It reaches the same conclusions and can be found in Appendix 1.

EFFECTIVENESS AND THE INDIVIDUAL DOCTOR

The literature review presented in Appendix 1, concludes that:

➤ Awareness has increased of the prevalence of self-directed learning among professionals and of the role this has to play in their ongoing development: most 'continuing learning' is likely to be initiated, organised, controlled and evaluated by the individual, and formal inputs play only a supporting, if important, role

➤ Evidence suggests that individual doctors vary considerably in their preference for different learning methods. These preferences must be taken into account rather than adopting a rigid view of how doctors 'ought' to like how to learn. Evidence suggests that a learning method is less important than many other factors.

Thus, any CPD system must allow the individual doctor to learn as that person wishes to learn. It should be 'catered towards individual learning needs and preferences'.[22] As Schostak *et al.*[8] point out:

> '... the literature stated that there was "no single, singular or correct way of doing CPD", and that the content, context and processes chosen were going to depend upon spheres of practice, learning styles and personal preferences.'

Their review reaches further conclusions that support the model of managed CPD put forward here:

> 'The evidence in the literature indicated that successful learning was much more likely to occur through active modes of learning than passive modes. This typically involved linking CPD with needs analysis assessments and the development of multiple learning activities. Furthermore, CPD was described as being at the heart of knowledge translation, bridging the transitions between theory and practice. Another recurrent theme, centred upon minimising the gap between theory and practice, was the principle of ensuring that knowledge does not remain abstract, i.e. as something that is learnt outside the practice arena. Thus, the literature recommended that effective knowledge should be integrated with

everyday working practices, and combined with follow-up activities in order to ensure reinforcement and critical development.'

We must conclude, therefore, that an evidence-based, managed approach to CPD, managing it as a creditable process, rather than attempting to define measurable units of activity with no known practical effect, complies with all good principles of regulation, education, and professional development and practice.

Implementing managed CPD

STEP ONE: IDENTIFY WHAT TO LEARN

Here we present the methods which can be used to help doctors identify what it is that they need or want to learn. Earlier, this step was presented as follows:

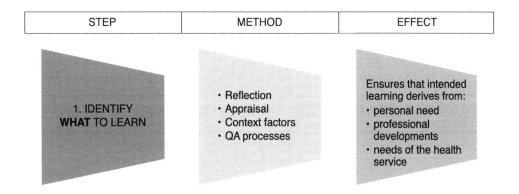

STEP	METHOD	EFFECT

1. IDENTIFY **WHAT** TO LEARN

- Reflection
- Appraisal
- Context factors
- QA processes

Ensures that intended learning derives from:
- personal need
- professional developments
- needs of the health service

To identify methods of ascertaining what to learn, we gathered those listed in the literature, by medical Royal Colleges and similar organisations. We also spoke with a sample of doctors about how they actually decided what to learn until no further ideas were contributed.

However, the demands of regulation and transparency require that doctors not only reflect on their learning needs and wants, but that this should also be done consciously and recorded. We therefore recommend that:

➤ The identification of learning needs/wants should occur within an appraisal or a professional conversation with a peer
➤ The process and its outcome should be recorded.

The appraisal might occur on an annual basis, or more frequently, if required.

> Appendix 2 presents a template record form for the appraisal or professional conversation session at which the doctor's learning needs or wants are identified and recorded.

HOW CAN LEARNING NEEDS BE IDENTIFIED?

Learning needs identification can be seen as a formal process or can be an integrated part of professional life.

However, Grant (2000)[23] points out that:

➤ Exclusive reliance on formal needs assessment could render education an instrumental and narrow process, rather than a creative, professional one

➤ Different learning methods tend to suit different doctors with different identified learning needs

➤ Doctors already use a wide range of formal and informal ways to identify their own learning needs as part of their ordinary practice

➤ These should be the starting point for designing formalised educational systems for professional improvement.

There is no commonly accepted definition of an educational need. Whole books are devoted to what an educational need might or might not be and what methods may be used to identify it. In the end, the methods used are simply a reflection of the view that is adopted about what an educational need actually is for the learner in question. The answer will be different for different learners. Norman[24] points out that:

> 'Learning needs are personal, specific, and identified by the individual learner through practice experience, reflection, questioning, practice audits, self-assessment tests, peer review, and other sources.'

He further suggests:

➤ Traditional approaches to continuing education that rely on self-assessment and self-learning are likely to be ineffective

➤ Centralised methods, such as regular relicensure or recertification examinations, are difficult to tailor to the characteristics of individual practices and are perceived as threatening.

The Good CPD Guide takes the view that methods of needs assessment for CPD must be appropriate to the characteristics of the profession and that it must be a part of the managed process of CPD. Needs assessment should be based in, and grow out of, professional practice.

In these times of transparency and accountability, there is sometimes a feeling that needs assessment should be done 'objectively' by an outside or independent agent. There is talk of doctors only being able to identify their educational 'wants' rather than their actual 'needs' (as though wanting something actually excludes the possibility that one might need it too!). It is often said that, given a free hand, doctors will only attend those educational events that concern things they already know and are interested in, rather than choosing the more challenging areas that are new to them. The evidence for such statements is rarely available.

The Good CPD Guide takes a different view of needs assessment, proposing that it is best seen as the result of three complementary processes:

➤ The professional practice of the doctor
➤ More formal processes such as audit or peer review
➤ The standards and plans of the health service in which the doctor works.

There are many ways doctors can identify their learning needs in relation to these three processes. Some of these are presented below.

SHOULD ALL CPD BE BASED ON SPECIFIC LEARNING NEEDS?

Although *The Good CPD Guide* describes methods of needs assessment, this is not to suggest that all professional learning should be based on specifically identified needs. Indeed, professional learning is often aimed at general development or reinforcement of knowledge and skills. Given that major characteristics of professional practice are its unpredictability and the unique nature of each professional encounter, to base all education on known needs would be highly counter-productive and unprofessional. There must be a balance of general professional CPD and CPD which is aimed at specific needs or outcomes:

➤ General professional CPD might be, for example, attendance at an international meeting for general updating purposes
➤ CPD aimed at specific needs might be, for example, learning a new technique or skill, or making up for some identified deficit.

Both types of CPD are required.

> Most of the methods listed simply occur as part of the normal routine of working. Some require a special effort to be made. Both approaches to educational needs assessment are acceptable and important. They form parts of professional behaviour.

The methods of needs identification described here, and gathered from the literature and reference to doctors' own experiences will enable a balance of both types of CPD. It is a balance that must be maintained.

HOW DO DOCTORS IDENTIFY THEIR LEARNING NEEDS?

This section lists the many ways doctors either identify a need or want to learn more. The list was compiled from the literature, by the hospital departments and consultants involved in the research project, and by the original *Good CPD Guide* authors.

However, identification of educational needs as a routine part of everyday professional practice is perhaps not quite enough these days. It is necessary to state how those needs were identified and to do that more consciously. This simply demands the awareness that needs are being identified and putting together a learning and follow-up plan which does something about them.

When planning CPD, doctors should be able, allowed and encouraged to cite any of the methods listed in this section (or others, if necessary) as the reason for wanting to undertake the CPD requested. Perhaps a balance of formal and informal methods would be desirable, but the main point is to demonstrate that a needs assessment or reflection has occurred and that the CPD planned is a rational choice.

There are many ways in which an individual's needs might be assessed. An appraisal or professional conversation with an appropriate colleague is an essential part of the way in which individual, departmental and other needs may be reflected on and planned for. This has been dealt with separately above, in relation to appraisal. The actual approaches to needs assessment, which might be reported in the appraisal meeting, are now presented in the following six groups:

➤ The clinician's own experience in direct patient care
➤ Interactions within the clinical team and department
➤ Non-clinical activities
➤ Formal approaches to audit and risk assessment
➤ Specific activities directed at needs assessment
➤ Peer review.

These methods of needs assessment are listed in Appendix 3.

NEEDS ASSESSMENT BASED ON THE CLINICIAN'S OWN EXPERIENCES IN DIRECT PATIENT CARE

TYPE	METHOD
The clinician's own experiences in direct patient care	➤ Blind spots ➤ Clinically-generated unknowns ➤ Competence standards ➤ Diaries ➤ Difficulties arising in practice ➤ Innovations in practice ➤ Knowledgeable patients ➤ Mistakes ➤ Other disciplines ➤ Patients' complaints and feedback ➤ Post-mortems and the clinico-pathological conference (CPC) ➤ The patient's unmet needs and the doctor's educational needs (PUNs and DENs) ➤ Reflection on practical experience

Blind spots

Often, long and detailed reflection on practice is not required to know that some further education or training might be in order. Technical and knowledge deficiencies, in particular, may suddenly and obviously be identified during the course of daily practice. These should be deliberately noted and plans for appropriate training made.

Clinically-generated unknowns

From time to time every doctor will encounter a clinical picture, reaction or process which is entirely unfamiliar. In such circumstances, the doctor must decide whether to refer the patient to another specialist or to find out about the observed phenomenon, or do both. In referring, it is likely that the doctor will learn about the entity from the colleague whose opinion is sought. There are many ways of dealing with such events and the choice is a matter of clinical judgment. The educational effect should be noted and recorded as a valid method of professional learning.

Competence standards

There are many worries that competence standards set a minimum level of performance that will limit people's aspirations for excellence.[25] Nonetheless, standards are necessary and so some societies, colleges and organisations have set them out, for example, in relation to minimal access therapy and other procedures. These may well prove to be very helpful as a baseline against which to assess (but not limit) one's own achievements. They could be a useful starting point for 'Gap Analysis' (*see* below).

Diaries

Keeping a diary of day-to-day events, especially critical incidents and difficulties, can help doctors reflect on why they have approached practical problems in particular ways and stimulate them to think of other avenues of approach. Looking back over a few months, it may be possible to detect certain patterns of behaviour, to think strategically about what may be achieved in future and take steps to acquire related CPD. Even if the diary is kept only for short spells, every now and then, it can help enable the writer to adopt a more reflective and strategic way of thinking that continues over time. Nowadays, a diary may be kept electronically. For example, the Canadian MOCOMP2 (Maintenance of Competence) procedure* involved logging queries and difficulties that arise in daily practice and, following the necessary reflection or research, noting 'solutions' alongside. Analysis of this record over time to reveal patterns, may also be conducted electronically. If a 'cluster' of queries emerges concerning treatments

*See Appendix 1 literature overview.

of diabetes, for example, this may indicate the need for more thorough on-going CPD activity in that area. A similar process can be undertaken simply with pen and paper.

Difficulties arising in practice

Difficulties arising in day-to-day practice are not always easy to identify, even when a system for doing so (such as adverse event reporting systems) is followed – and it is notoriously hard to spot one's own mistakes. They are often picked up by colleagues (nurses, junior doctors, peers), through audit procedures, during discussions and sometimes, as a result of complaint or disaster. No doubt doctors try to analyse errors and difficulties of all types in order to overcome them; related CPD activity may well help them do so.

Innovations in practice

Any doctor who thinks for a moment, will be able to list many ways in which his or her practice has changed both over the years and also recently. Practice changes constantly. New drugs, advancing technology and equipment, new methods, procedures and techniques are always being introduced. Along with these comes the need to learn to use each of them properly and well. Acquiring the training or education to do so should be a high priority and properly planned.

Knowledgeable patients

In these days of information from the internet, patient-orientated charities and in magazines and libraries, many patients become highly knowledgeable about the disorders that they or members of their family might have. Some patients will turn up to the clinic already informed about what they think might be their diagnosis. Others learn as the condition develops. It is not unknown for patients to appear with articles from highly technical medical journals. Patients also can belong to self-help and support groups that are valuable sources of information to them. Doctors recognise patients as valuable sources of education and knowledge but such patients can also highlight areas about which the doctor needs to become more informed. The doctor must always be in a position to discuss with patients the knowledge that they bring and assess it.

Mistakes

When a clinical mistake has occurred, this can be a trigger for individual reflection and identification of learning needs, as well as organisational review. Not all errors are a result of the doctor's deficiencies. Sometimes the context is the culprit. An analysis of the reason for the mistake must be made. For example, was the mistake due to:

➤ Lack of knowledge?
➤ Overwork and stress?

➤ Inadequate protocols or guidance?
➤ Contextual issues?

When a need is identified in this way, appropriate learning can be planned and fed back into practice in the most effective way. If the mistake was the doctor's, the organisational climate must be such as to allow the admission that this was the case.

Other disciplines

Doctors work with other disciplines in many contexts: clinical work, committees, management roles, and so on. Every discipline has its own knowledge, concepts, skills and models of practice. Sometimes, some of these will be of relevance to medical practice and will either 'make you think' or be worth enquiring into further, especially if it is an area which appears to have relevance for medical practice.

Patients' complaints and feedback

Patients' views on all aspects of their experience of healthcare are offered increasingly frequently and also solicited by hospitals and general practices. Often, complaints are about waiting times and other aspects of the service administration. However, they may also call into question a doctor's clinical skills or professional demeanour. These complaints can point to the need for particular kinds of CPD activity – which, in some cases, the hospital, department or practice may want to encourage or even insist upon. Furthermore, regular review of patients' complaints and feedback can be undertaken, forming an important part of formal CPD planning, as well as a source for the individual doctor's own plans.

Post-mortems and the clinico-pathological conference (CPC)

Discussions between the clinician and pathologist can be a fruitful source of identifying learning needs for both.

PUNs and DENs[26]

This method has been developed and used in general practice.
➤ PUNs = Patient unmet needs
➤ DENs = Doctor educational needs

Richard Eve from Taunton, who developed the PUNs approach, recommends that a doctor collects PUNs during a set number of surgeries (outpatients, ward rounds, lists) simply by asking after each patient or session: 'Was I equipped to meet the patient's needs? Could I have done better?' A note should be made of the answer to these questions: these will be the PUNs. In this way, an area or areas will be identified that might benefit from further learning or development: these will be the DENs. Eve points out that some PUNs will not be met by education but by changes elsewhere, such as in organisation, or administration. For CPD, it is necessary to identify those PUNs which truly indicate a DEN and then act on them.

Reflection on practical experience

Day-to-day practice or teaching, in clinics, on the ward and in the operating theatre typically throws up queries and difficulties that must be resolved. Reflecting on these experiences can alert doctors to the need for some reading on a particular topic, the need to attend a course, or undertake some more systematic research. The process of reflecting on practice may be more or less deliberate and formal. Doctors might:

> Simply jot down a few notes in a diary after a tricky consultation, to be followed up later
> Team up with a colleague to talk about recent experiences in clinical practice and draw out CPD implications
> Discuss practical issues and proposals for CPD during an appraisal meeting.

INTERACTIONS WITHIN THE CLINICAL TEAM AND DEPARTMENT

TYPE	*METHOD*
Interactions within the clinical team and department	> Clinical meetings: departmental and grand rounds > Department business plan > Department educational meetings > External recruitment > Junior staff > Management roles > Mentoring

Both hospital consultants and general practitioners work within a clinical team. For many hospital-based doctors, the individual clinical department is the core unit within which they work while, for others, the clinical team may be the source of most contact with others. For all clinicians, interactions with the clinical team or the clinical department may be important in indicating educational needs.

Clinical meetings: departmental and grand rounds

Educational needs are often identified in the course of events that are primarily designed to offer education or to review practice. Departmental clinical meetings and grand rounds are such occasions where cases or some aspects of practice are discussed and everyone learns something. However, such meetings, by their very nature, can also leave participants with areas that they still need to learn more about or acquire some skill in. A major part of learning is the discovery that there is always more to learn!

Department business plan

Managed CPD must integrate the learning needs of the individual doctor and the requirements of the service. From time to time, the clinical department's development priorities may influence consultants' or GPs' decisions about appropriate CPD activity. For example, new management tasks may emerge or its members may wish to introduce a new clinical service or technique which will involve attending a training course or visiting a similar department elsewhere. All such developments will be represented in the department's business plan, which is the subject of negotiation with senior staff. The business plan should be taken into account during negotiations about CPD plans. To aid this process, in meetings where the business plan is discussed, doctors will need to take account of its implications for their own CPD plans.

Department educational meetings

At these meetings, usually held weekly, clinical topics that affect the whole department are discussed. In hospitals, the discussion may be led by a consultant, or by a doctor in training whose knowledge of a particular aspect of the specialty curriculum has recently been called upon, challenged or enlarged through the demands of clinical practice. In primary care, this may be a GP, the registrar or another member of the primary care team. Such discussion of the interface between theory and practice, and of up-to-date experience in the field, may raise awareness of ground that needs to be explored further and indicate an appropriate area for CPD.

External recruitment

New members of staff joining a clinical team invariably bring with them the ideas and skills they have acquired in previous jobs. If they are encouraged to share their experience (rather than required to conform to the team's regular practices as soon as possible) then such 'new blood' can act as a stimulus, helping to revitalise the team. In the process, its existing members may discover aspects of knowledge and skill that need development through CPD.

Junior staff

Senior doctors value junior doctors for the different range of knowledge and skills which they may possess and especially for their capacity to ask questions and challenge accepted thinking. Interactions with junior doctors may well indicate areas that need to be followed up.

Management roles

Many doctors today become involved in management. They may be clinical directors, medical directors or involved in other aspects of the management of the health service. New roles bring new learning needs and will often be accompanied by the possibility of training. Before taking up such training, some thought should be given to exactly what training is required and what the priorities for training are.

Mentoring[27]

Mentors are usually more senior colleagues, or those with particular expertise in appropriate areas, who operate 'outside' the formal structures and hierarchy of the organisation. They normally offer one or more of three main services:
➤ emotional and psychological support
➤ direct assistance with career and professional development
➤ role modelling.

Even if there is no recognised system of mentoring in a hospital or practice, doctors may act as mentors to each other, including those of the same 'rank' – for example, a doctor may team up with a colleague, agreeing to meet for discussion at regular intervals and to observe each other in action from time to time. In the case of mentoring between equals, where no senior/junior or career guidance elements are involved, colleagues can be more constructively critical of each other's knowledge and performance, and so help one another identify areas of CPD need.

NEEDS ASSESSMENT BASED ON THE CLINICIAN'S NON-CLINICAL ACTIVITIES

TYPE	*METHOD*
Non-clinical activities	➤ Academic activities ➤ Conferences ➤ International visits ➤ Journal articles ➤ Medico-legal cases ➤ Press and media ➤ Professional conversations ➤ Research ➤ Teaching

Clinicians undertake many non-clinical activities in administration, planning, leading and managing the team as well as rotas or schedules. Many of these provide a springboard to further learning.

Academic activities

Many consultants regard such tasks as refereeing a journal article or research proposal, or acting as an examiner, simply as part of the job. However, the reading, discussion or observation involved can reveal gaps in the doctor's knowledge or give rise to new areas of interest to be followed up. Getting into the habit of jotting down ideas picked up from such activities in a notebook or on a palm-top computer, along with associated references and further thoughts may, over time, yield a fruitful agenda for a period of CPD study.

Conferences

Participating in a conference is usually seen as a way of learning and keeping up to date, but such meetings can also be a rich source of ideas for appropriate CPD activity. The conference programme alone provides a convenient, up-to-date listing of topics of current interest in the specialty, acting as a kind of 'consciousness raiser'. This list may then be fleshed out by abstracts, talks, demonstrations, and conference papers. Furthermore, conferences offer the opportunity to meet many national and international colleagues, and to discuss issues of mutual interest informally. Such talk, both formal and informal, may alert participants to deficits in their knowledge or inspire them to explore new avenues of practice and enquiry through CPD.

International visits

Visits to colleagues overseas, such as the travelling clubs organised by many specialties, may reveal areas of deficit in specialist knowledge or skill and even introduce the doctor to new ideas and procedures that give rise to subsequent CPD. An international visit may also provide the kind of break from routine that enables doctors to 'distance' themselves from their day-to-day work and gain a new perspective on it. Such a mind-broadening experience may make a particularly stimulating CPD activity for doctors in the mid-to-late career stages.

Journal articles

The wealth of information which surrounds a practising clinician can itself prompt a need to learn more. Journal articles and other written materials can often highlight a relevant area of knowledge about which more information or experience is required. Such information sources are triggers to self-assessment of educational need – although we very rarely think of them in those terms as it is all a normal part of professional life. Since reading is one of the most important ways doctors have of keeping up to date, it is hardly surprising that through reading doctors can also find out what more they have to learn.

Medico-legal cases

Being an expert witness or being otherwise involved in medico-legal cases causes a doctor to think about clinical medicine in ways that are different from that required for daily clinical practice. Lawyers will want to know about detail, derivation, evidence, underlying basic science, the basis of clinical judgment, exceptions, related cases and conditions, thinking processes, related clinical skills, the health services context and many other aspects of a case. Preparation for medico-legal cases not only reveals areas that require some further personal education, but also will cause the doctor to acquire that education very quickly indeed!

Press and media

Doctors may need to undertake certain CPD activities associated with cases reported in the press or on television, which prompt enquiries from patients, such as 'scares' about the effects of contraceptive pills and HRT on women or developments in research into the causes of sudden infant death. The release of new drugs tends to arouse particularly intense interest, especially when they may affect large numbers of people; for example, the advent of Prozac for the treatment of depression and of Viagra for impotence in men. Any developments in treatment for cancers and HIV/AIDS, or even rumours of them, can also be expected to give rise to intense speculation, confusion, raised hopes and anxiety. Generally, doctors need to be aware of current press and media preoccupations and, in some cases, undertake CPD in order to keep abreast of developments – not least to be able to inform and reassure their patients.

Professional conversations

Clinicians live in a rich daily professional learning environment which is dominated by discussion of patients and practice. Doctors discuss their own patients with other doctors whose views are sought. They discuss shared patients and others' patients and experiences. These informal professional conversations are as much a part of learning and of identifying learning needs as any other type of more formal approach to needs assessment. Such professional conversations contain feedback on performance in relation to specific patients when the management or outcome of treatment is discussed. They also contain new learning and open up new areas for learning which are often followed up quite deliberately. Where this is so, a learning need has been identified in a relevant and professional manner.

Research

Clearly, doctors' own research preferences and projects give rise to the need for certain challenging CPD activities, such as studying relevant journal articles and writing and publishing papers. Researchers will no doubt also need to attend courses, whether in the substantive area of research or in research design, methods, funding and management. The hospital and clinical department (and perhaps primary care groups) have an interest in supporting all CPD proposals related to doctors' research, since research output contributes to the academic reputation of the hospital/department/practice and the funds available to it. So when planning and designing research projects, doctors should aim to identify those CPD activities and courses that will enable them to do their work well, or better.

Teaching

Teaching in classrooms, seminars, the operating theatre and on ward rounds is usually regarded as 'part of the job', like the other academic activities doctors perform regularly. Yet both preparing for teaching and the activity itself are fertile sources of insight into doctors' own educational needs. It would be surprising if the reading and thinking involved, and the challenge of student questioning, did not reveal some gaps in doctors' knowledge and experience, aspects of the subject that may be glossed over, and relevant skills in need of some honing. Such lacunae, duly noted down, might amount to a personalised 'refresher course' to be followed through during a period of CPD study leave.*

FORMAL APPROACHES TO QUALITY MANAGEMENT AND RISK ASSESSMENT

TYPE	METHOD
Formal approaches to quality management and risk assessment	➤ Audit ➤ Morbidity patterns ➤ Patient adverse events ➤ Patient satisfaction surveys ➤ Risk assessment ➤ Portfolios

There are many initiatives directed at either quality management or the management of medico-legal risk. All of these may provide an indication of educational need.

Audit

Medical and clinical audit are by now well-established in primary and secondary care, although perhaps not as well used to identify educational needs as had first been intended. Nonetheless, it might be worth doing one of two things:
➤ Look at the results of on-going audits and analyse whether or not there are any obvious educational implications of the issues raised
➤ Design new audits that directly tackle areas in which you suspect there might be a case for further education – for example, in techniques or treatments.

---

*If your organisation does not have a study leave application form, one is suggested in Appendix 4.

Guidelines on the formal use of audit for educational purposes are available elsewhere.[28]

Morbidity patterns

Patterns of illness and disease in the patient population served should be a prime source of indicators for CPD. Epidemiological data can also be used to enable the doctor to reflect on personal strengths, weaknesses and interests when planning what CPD will be undertaken. Such patterns can and do change over time with social and societal changes and with changes in treatments, so a review of morbidity patterns should be undertaken at intervals to determine what aspects the doctor might wish to learn more about.

Patient adverse events

Adverse event screening is a typical method of audit and sometimes it will be useful as a method of educational needs assessment. However, the results of such screening might also have implications which concern organisation, management and other factors beyond the skills, attitudes or knowledge of the clinician. So the results of adverse event surveys should always be looked at closely to determine whether an underlying educational deficit or need is evident.

Patient satisfaction surveys

Surveys can be used to gain feedback from users or potential users about the care or service offered. A survey of a particular group of patients might supply the most appropriate information. When undertaking a patient satisfaction survey, the objective should be focused and clearly defined. Patient satisfaction surveys can probably only deal with a very limited set of objectives that are relevant to a doctor's educational needs but, nonetheless, can be valuable in areas such as communication and information as well as finding out more about specific outcomes. Patient satisfaction is now also an integral part of the clinical effectiveness limb of the clinical governance agenda.

Risk assessment

Risk assessment is now a usual part of service management. It is closely related not only to how that service is best managed but also to how doctors make decisions about diagnosis, treatment and care, to how resources are allocated and how junior doctors are trained and supervised. The risk assessment function can reveal doctors' own educational needs from two points of view:

➤ First, doctors will be asked to contribute to the assessment of risk, in which case recourse to research evidence, as well as accumulated experience might be necessary

➤ Second, the risk assessment policies which the service adopts locally will cause doctors to assure themselves of their correctness – in which case, some further personal education may well be in order.

Portfolios

Many professional organisations and regulatory authorities now offer or demand portfolios, most commonly online, in which a doctor deposits evidence of both practice and education. It has been said that[29] the possible benefits of portfolios include:

➤ The potential to evaluate a doctor's ability to reflect on practice and learn from experience

➤ Improved patient care (based on the evidence that, where properly used, portfolios can enhance learning from experience and lead to improved patient care)

➤ The flexibility to demonstrate professional development over time as well as contemporaneous satisfactory performance

➤ Ability to be tailored to an individual's practice profile and their contents determined by a doctor's own learning/practice needs.

SPECIFIC ACTIVITIES DIRECTED AT NEEDS ASSESSMENT

TYPE	METHOD
Specific activities directed at needs assessment	➤ Critical incident surveys ➤ Gap analysis ➤ Objective tests of knowledge and skill ➤ Observation ➤ Revalidation systems ➤ Self-assessment ➤ Video assessment of performance

This group of activities contains a series of well-described approaches to needs assessment that may become more widespread as regulation and governance increase.

Critical incident surveys

Although critical incident studies are most well-known for purposes of research, the technique can equally be used to help individuals identify their own learning needs. The method has a well-established pedigree deriving from its use in a study of aircrews during World War II. It has since been used to identify competencies (and incompetencies) in many professions. Critical incident review is best undertaken with a colleague or appraiser. The technique involves the doctor in describing a number of incidents in his or her own recent practice which are examples of good and poor practice. Each incident should be well-described in terms of exactly what happened and its outcome. In conversation, the doctor and colleague/appraiser should analyse what it was about the incident that made it good or poor practice. If this is done with a number of incidents, a picture of both the doctor's strengths and educational needs can be derived. There is a large amount of literature which describes various detailed approaches to critical incident analysis but this general approach will be sufficient for purposes of identifying learning needs for CPD.

Gap analysis

Gap analysis is based on the idea that a learning need is the gap between current and ideal performance. Gap analysis is undertaken by:

➤ Defining the knowledge, skills, attitudes or competencies which are required to perform the relevant role excellently

➤ Defining where the person is in relation to each aspect defined. This can be done either individually or with the help of others.

A numerical or descriptive rating scale, properly piloted, can be used. For example:

Ability to perform a transoesophageal echocardiogram	Not achieved	Partially achieved	Almost achieved	Fully achieved

The doctor can then concentrate continuing education activity on those items which display the greatest discrepancy between achieved and desired competencies. Gap analysis can be undertaken by means of questionnaires, interviews, audit of records, standardised patients and clinical stimulated-recall interviews and so on. However, these are formal methods that might be inappropriate to the professional context of CPD. This method is often used where norms and standards are already defined. The approach has several potential disadvantages. It can miss the less easily defined, but equally important areas and tends to reduce needs assessment to a simplistic, non-analytical and mechanical process. However, as a broad indication of need, it may well have some use.

Objective tests of knowledge and skill

Objective tests of knowledge and skill rarely impinge on the life of a doctor once all the qualifying examinations have been passed. After that stage, reflection or feedback on practice, in one form or another, with or without the assistance of a peer, become the predominant modes of assessment of need to learn. Nonetheless, objective tests are sometimes made available by professional organisations as part of specific courses, and by commercial publishing companies and journals. Computer-based tests are also available in some specialties in the form of multiple-choice questions, patient management problems, and so on. Such tests might not always have been developed with the psychometric rigour that should characterise undergraduate and postgraduate examinations, but they still might prove to be useful in highlighting areas of knowledge or skill that are in need of attention. Of course, with such tests, the agenda is set by the test producer, not by the test-taker and the areas covered might be relatively small and perhaps not closely related to the central concerns of the doctor taking the test. It is for the individual to make that judgment and use the tests and their results accordingly. If a specific area of knowledge or skill needs to be rigorously tested, then it is possible to develop objective tests of many types. but, in general, these do not seem to be suited to the purpose of identifying learning needs for CPD.

Observation

Observation of clinical practice, in the sense of working alongside and informally judging performance, has been an important tool in medical education for many years. It is one that has been formalised and refined for higher specialist training by a number of colleges. It can also be used very effectively as part of a peer review process for doctors contributing towards their CPD plans. Observation is probably best suited to procedural, technical and other demonstrable skills and physical tasks, communication and interpersonal skills. It is probably insufficient on its own for looking at thought processes and the clinical reasoning involved in case management. An advantage of real time observation is that it can potentially make useful judgments about what the doctor can do in the real world, with real patients. It can be fitted into normal working hours without detriment to the service. Feedback can be given immediately and plans for CPD made. Unstructured observation does not easily meet the necessary criteria of validity and reliability that assessment in other circumstances might require. Nonetheless, for purposes of helping a doctor to identify areas of practice that would benefit from CPD, observation can be useful. This is especially so if it is repeated on more than one occasion by more than one observer, and if it is also followed by a discussion of what the observer has noted. The assessment of learning needs is not the exact science that the assessment of learning aspires to be. Given this, observation is worth considering among the panoply of peer review instruments.

Revalidation systems

Although revalidation is not, at the time of writing, a fact of professional life in medicine, such systems, should they arrive, may well set standards and define what it is that a senior doctor should be able to do, know and display. It is perhaps both a positive and negative thing that such standards might exclusively drive the CPD agenda for many doctors. On the one hand, such processes will ensure minimal standards of safe practice. On the other hand, they may also discourage excellence and narrow professional horizons unless they are very carefully formulated. Of course, revalidation might not set standards for performance, but might simply state that needs must be identified, in which case, the listing here might prove to be useful.

Self-assessment

Self-assessment of learning needs takes many forms, ranging from informal and opportunistic reflection on practice to highly-structured and formal processes. Current practice across all professions suggests that responsibility for planning and undertaking continuing education rests with the individual professional. However, finding the time and personal motivation to identify one's own learning needs is often a challenge. Consequently, various formal systems and self-assessments have been developed, often by professional organisations, for helping individuals to think about their experience, identify the need to acquire knowledge, skills or experience, and plan ways of fulfilling these needs.

It should be emphasised that self-assessment of learning needs in the professional context generally refers to some form of reflecting on practice, rather than formal assessment of knowledge, skills and attitudes using a well-developed test instrument. However, self-assessment alone is possibly not a powerful method. As Regher and Eva state[30]

> 'To be effectively self-regulating, the profession generally depends on the individual practitioner to self-regulate his own maintenance of competence activities. This model of individual self-regulation, in turn, depends on the practitioner's ability to self-assess gaps in competence and willingness to seek out opportunities to redress these gaps when identified. The literature relevant to these processes, however, would suggest this model of individual self-regulation is overly optimistic.'

When combined with other methods, however, this criticism may well be attenuated.

Video assessment of performance

This is both a learning method and a way of identifying educational needs. It is fully described as a learning method under Step Two. The use of video-recorded performance to identify learning needs involves the following steps:

➤ Production of a video tape of a real (or perhaps simulated) performance – for example, a consultation

➤ Reviewing the tape with others or against defined criteria and standards of good practice in the area

➤ Noting any areas which require development, remediation, education or training.

It is often the case that when the video is reviewed the problem areas will not only be identified but also discussed and dealt with as part of the same process. However, it might be the case that some areas of practice would benefit from education or training in another context. In this case, the video will be used only for identification of learning needs and for planning what education is required.

PEER REVIEW

TYPE	METHOD
Peer review	➤ External peer review ➤ Informal peer review of the individual doctor ➤ Internal peer review ➤ Multidisciplinary peer review ➤ Physician assessment (360 degree assessment, multisource feedback)

Peer review is a generic term which covers many formal and informal activities involving doctors assessing one another's practice, and giving feedback and perhaps advice about possible education and training strategies to tackle any problems identified. Peer review is usually conducted by a pair or small group of doctors according to a focused agenda that might be broad or relatively constrained. Peer review can be conducted with greater or lesser degrees of formality but some kind of report or agreement would be expected at the end of the process to document what was found and concluded. Peer review is dealt with as a method of needs assessment, as a learning method and as a means of following-up of CPD. There are many types of peer review and all types can serve all these purposes.

External peer review

External peer review involves review by a visiting group or individual. It is a system for managing the quality of professional work. Part of such management clearly involves an evaluation of the benefits of CPD. Peer review also holds out the prospect of identifying deficiencies and therefore identifying needs for CPD. Clearly the scope of the process extends well beyond CPD. External peer review provides a national benchmark for the delivery of all forms of specialist care. It is a valid method of demonstrating professional self-regulation. External peer review is designed to be appropriate across all specialties. The peer review should take place on a regular, perhaps five-yearly, basis. It is also suitable for alternating with internal peer review.

External peer review has a number of advantages. The approval of peers is excellent for morale. At the same time, the visitors can identify areas of practice where there may be room for improvement, and therefore identify the learning needs of the doctor or the team. The method is as applicable to the peripatetic locum doctor and to the isolated community-based psychiatrist as it is to the cardiologists in a tertiary referral centre or GPs in the community.

Peer review of the team can be less threatening than peer review of the individual. While the members of the team may 'stand back-to-back' when being interviewed, it becomes clear when the visitors interview the managers, the nurses and others, if one of the team members is performing less satisfactorily than the others. By involving members of a team that has been recently visited and a team that is to be visited in the near future, every team not only has ownership of the exercise, but also gets the opportunity to visit two other teams in the five-year cycle. Such visits therefore have educational value in that the visitors learn how others do things differently.

But there are some disadvantages. It is expensive. For example, one European scheme involves three visitors, who must be trained, in a total of 58 hours of work. Before a visit, a questionnaire about the team's workload, facilities, CPD activities and audit activities is completed. In addition, the visitors obtain relevant information from the national statistics (for example, the number of hysterectomies done in the locality per annum per 100 000 population). During the six-hour visit, the team is interviewed, managers, nurses and local GPs are interviewed, the facilities and a random selection of case notes are inspected. Immediate feedback is given to the team and a report is subsequently produced. The method depends on every doctor belonging to a team. As the visitors are all from one specialty, they may not be optimally equipped to assess the generalist skills and knowledge of the team. Inclusion of a questionnaire about individual team members is probably inappropriate, because a team-based peer review does not permit a confidential discussion of the responses to a questionnaire about individuals.

Informal peer review of the individual doctor

Informal systems of peer review are quite common. For example, consultants carry out combined clinics, colleagues discuss the management of cases in clinical meetings, and systems of internal referral within hospitals all form a background against which internal informal peer review may take place. These diverse processes may contribute to the assessment of need for CPD of the team or the individual doctor.

Wherever there is peer review, there is the opportunity for assessment of learning needs. There are many other ways in which informal peer review is already in place in hospitals. They include:

➤ Seeking a second opinion about a patient. This acknowledges that the person seeking the second opinion recognises the limitations of his or her knowledge or skills. The person providing the second opinion (the 'expert') can help educate the referring doctor and clearly gains insight into the state of knowledge of the referring doctor. The roles of expert and referring doctor are often reversed in different clinical situations

➤ Many consultants undertake combined clinics with a colleague from another specialty

➤ Departmental meetings with case presentations also provide an opportunity for informal peer review which may reveal learning needs.

The process might be extended to include:

➤ Sharing ward rounds. Two doctors in the same specialty may share a ward round on a regular (although not necessarily frequent) basis. They can then comment on the management of each other's patients. If conducted in an atmosphere of openness and trust, this can be a valuable educational exercise and stimulate the identification of further learning needs. Scoring points against each other will terminate this activity

➤ Outpatient activity with combined clinics or the discussion of the management of patients from clinics.

Internal peer review

Internal peer review is a process that enables the individual doctor to manage his/her CPD. It can involve the doctor, team, employer and both the professional body and the training provider. It is similar to the process of managed CPD itself.

The role of the individual doctor in identifying learning needs is to:

➤ Assess his/her own current knowledge, personal qualities and skills

➤ Review with the other members of the clinical team, to identify the knowledge and skills the team and the individual need to meet the business plan of the organisation

➤ Identify, prioritise and record the learning needs.

The record of the doctor's learning needs, development plan and achievement can be paper-based, but software is also commercially and commonly available, especially in the form of an electronic portfolio. The method is applicable to anyone who works in a team or an organisation.

It has advantages. The process formalises the identification of learning needs. Once this step has been undertaken, it becomes possible to make a judgment about whether those needs have been met. In addition, the formal process may improve the quality of CPD because individuals plan what they need to do to improve the care of their patients. Thus, the CPD is directed towards the needs of the individual, the team and the organisation with the goal of improving the care of patients. The training provider can prioritise the development of training courses and materials based on the sample of Personal Development Plans.

But there are disadvantages:

➤ The method is crucially dependent on doctors recording their development needs and achievements

➤ A number of individuals may spend some time in the process of review of an individual clinician which makes the process expensive.

Multidisciplinary peer review

It is possible for other professions to help doctors identify learning needs. In some specialties, this is a routine occurrence. For example, pathology laboratories are subject to regular accreditation and review of all procedures and processes involving all staff: technicians, doctors and administrative and clerical. The process of preparing for accreditation involves discussion and review of practice with input on a multiprofessional basis. This can identify learning needs and actions to be taken before the review itself.

Multidisciplinary peer review is a wide-ranging quality assurance activity. The approach often requires that assessment be made by a number of health professionals from a range of disciplines by questionnaire. Each must be in a position to judge the performance of the doctor, and be prepared to complete ratings of various aspects of competence through a 360 degree process. Members of the multidisciplinary assessment team will vary according to the specialty of the doctor. For example, an orthopaedic surgeon might invite anaesthetists, rheumatologists, radiologists, operating theatre nurses, outpatient and ward nurses, local GPs and physiotherapists, as well as orthopaedic surgeon colleagues to complete a questionnaire.

A further questionnaire is then used to collect information from between 12 and 20 respondents and the results are pooled and collated. The questionnaire must be specially designed. The first step is to agree on the attributes or competencies to be assessed. Judgments are based on norms or agreed decision-making guidelines. Each item is related to a rating scale, the extremes of which are defined in terms of the highest and lowest levels of performance. The questionnaire must be pilot-tested before being introduced for general use. Completion of the rating form should take no longer than ten minutes if a satisfactory response rate is to be achieved.

The method can be used to help identify the strengths and weaknesses of an individual doctor. It is particularly valuable for gathering information on personal attributes, interpersonal and communication skills and teamwork.

The advantages are that the method is probably valid and reliable as long as 12 or more people respond to the questionnaire.

➤ A wide range of people can be consulted, including medical colleagues in the hospital, junior doctors, local GPs, nurses, physiotherapists and other colleagues.

➤ As long as confidentiality is maintained, the doctor can obtain helpful feedback on his/her performance.

The main disadvantage in using this method lies in determining the decision-making rules. The expense of multidisciplinary peer review is unlikely to be justified purely for the purpose of evaluating CPD needs. However, where the system is in place for quality control purposes it becomes a realistic possibility.

Physician assessment (360 degree assessment, multisource feedback)

This is a particular variant of peer review which was originated by the American Board of Internal Medicine[31] and further developed by the Royal Australasian College of Physicians. To undertake such an assessment, the doctor nominates a number of colleagues (for example, 15) to be assessors. Each is sent a standard rating form by the organising body (which could be the department, the trust or the college) and is asked to rate the doctor on various clinical skills, humanistic and other qualities. The ratings are fed back to the doctor who takes educational action accordingly. The system shows encouraging levels of validity, reliability and acceptability and has the advantage of credibility to the doctor who nominates personal assessors. This is otherwise known as 360 degree assessment,[32] or multisource feedback.[33]

STEP TWO: PLAN HOW TO LEARN — DOCUMENTATION

This second step in the process involves planning how to learn and recording that plan as part of the transparent, managed process. This step was presented above as follows:

STEP	METHOD	EFFECT

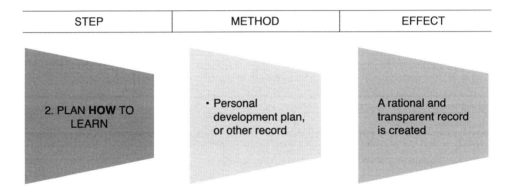

2. PLAN HOW TO LEARN — • Personal development plan, or other record — A rational and transparent record is created

Appraisal was presented in Step One as part of the means of identifying learning needs and wants. But the appraisal process also involves a record of the discussion and its conclusions. Part of that record addresses the learning plan and practical arrangements. There might also be an application for study leave. Appendices 2 and 4 suggest a format for the appraisal form and for a study leave application form.

The final document that might be required is a Personal Development Plan. This can be described as follows[*]:

> **Personal development planning** is the process of creating an action plan based on awareness, reflection, goal-setting and planning for personal development within the context of a career, education, or for self-improvement.

Personal Development Plans are now a widespread phenomenon in industry and the professions. In medicine, the most junior of trainees is guided to start

[*]http://en.wikipedia.org/wiki/Personal_development_planning

keeping such a document and lodging it in their portfolios, as this following guidance illustrates:

Your foundation school will provide you with the information you need on how to access your portfolio such as website address, log-in details and password. The exact format of each e-portfolio may vary but they generally include the following sections:
➤ Personal and Professional Development Plan (PDP)
➤ Meetings with your educational and clinical supervisors
➤ Workplace-based assessments
➤ Reflective reports and other evidence
➤ Sign-off documents.*

It is explained elsewhere that:

> PDPs are a means to identify educational need and to document and hence demonstrate that need has been addressed**.

Appendix 7 suggests a format for a Personal Development Plan.

Planning is therefore a process of undertaking and recording the steps of the CPD cycle. The documentation of this cycle is important both to guide the doctor and appraiser and for purposes of accountability and demonstration. In those countries where CPD is part of the job plan, of professional recognition or of continued registration (such as for revalidation in the UK), the documentation is a key element which might be represented as follows:

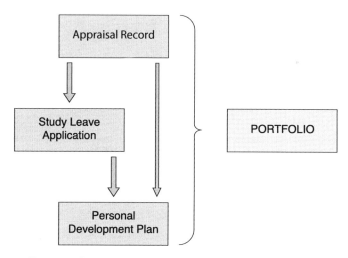

Figure 5: Documentation associated with the CPD cycle

*www.foundationprogramme.nhs.uk/pages/foundation-docs/e-portfolio
**www.patient.co.uk/doctor/Personal-Development-Plans.htm

A key part of planning how to learn is knowing what learning options are available. The next section describes the ways in which doctors do learn and we suggest that these should be recognised and built on.

STEP THREE: LEARN

Here we present the variety of learning methods that doctors can and do use to address their CPD learning needs and wants. The literature review shows clearly that there is no 'best learning method'. So here we present some of the very many ways in which doctors actually continue to learn. It is our view that all these should be acceptable within a CPD credit system that recognises the four-stage process rather than the learning method or isolated learning events. Earlier, this step was presented as follows:

STEP	METHOD	EFFECT

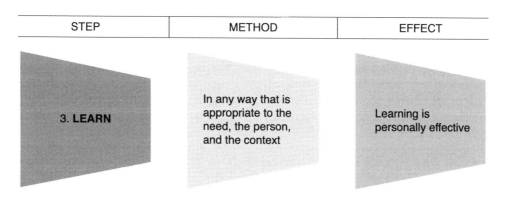

3. LEARN	In any way that is appropriate to the need, the person, and the context	Learning is personally effective

---

Although this section presents a variety of possible learning methods, we also assume that the learning method will be chosen, perhaps within an appraisal session, and then will be noted in the record, such as that presented in Appendix 2, or in an electronic portfolio or similar.

LEARNING IN A PROFESSION

Learning in a profession is quite unlike any other kind of learning. Doctors live in a rich learning environment, constantly involved in and surrounded by professional interaction and conversation, educational events, information and feedback. The search for the one best or 'right' way of learning is a counsel of despair, as the review of the effectiveness of CPD demonstrates (*see* Appendix 1). Professions are simply not amenable to that kind of educational confinement. The myriad research papers that try to discover how doctors learn show, at best, the complexity of the process.

One well-established finding is that multiple CPD interventions targeted at specific behaviour will result in positive change in that behaviour.[34] What those interventions are, is of less importance than their multiplicity and targeted nature. The system of managed CPD encourages targeted educational activity where that is appropriate.

When doctors identify a specific personal learning need, the wide range of preferred learning methods is also demonstrated. For example, in a study of 366 primary care physicians[35] who identified recent clinical problems which needed more knowledge or skill to solve, 55 different learning methods were selected. Problem-type turned out to be the major determinant of learning method in the practice setting.

Schostak *et al.* (2010)[12] also found a wide variety of learning methods in their sample of doctors:

'Recapping, the sheer variety of ways in which interviewees responded to the question: "How do you define effective CPD for you yourself?" covered a broad spectrum. This can be seen from the following selection of the very diverse range of responses:

➤ Moving people on through a mixture of employing the tools of learning, needs analysis and personal development plans
➤ Of experiencing a dissemination of new concepts because text books are typically five years out of date
➤ "Getting to know of developments within the NHS, particularly from a managerial point of view"
➤ It involves clinical management; learning about people management skills; about knowing oneself and one's limitations and attempting to address that
➤ Attendance at conferences, workshops
➤ Accumulation of credits
➤ The giving of presentations
➤ Reading
➤ Private study
➤ On-the-job learning
➤ Editing a journal
➤ Group-work
➤ Talking with colleagues and "corridor conversations"
➤ Meetings
➤ Ticking boxes
➤ Networking
➤ "Putting yourself next to people (so that) having recognised a weakness (…) you've put into place some ways of improving that"
➤ "Signing off"
➤ Promoting evidence-based medicine
➤ Learning to listen to the patient
➤ Knowing when to talk to the patient (child) or to the parents.

Such diversity must be read as a strong indication, supported by the literature review, that CPD is personal and owned by the individual.'

Under such recognised conditions, the idea of approving a CPD event might seem slightly incongruous.

So, there is no magic educational 'bullet'. Research even suggests that education is not a strong factor in changing clinicians' behaviour at all[36]. Where it is, medical journals, readings and scientific conferences are frequently cited as most effective. However, such discrete events and methods do not add up to the true picture of education and continuing learning in medicine. Doctors' learning is integrated with their practice and arises from it as much as it is separated from it. The style of integrated practice and learning develops during the successive stages of medical education and has been studied in other professions and trades. Such learning through practice is called 'situated learning'.[37]

Essentially, during the years of medical education, the learner moves the site of main learning from the necessary simulated, controlled and only peripherally professionally involved environment that is constructed during medical school, to the real environment of clinical practice until that real environment takes over as the main source of learning itself.

The components of apprenticeship learning in postgraduate training have been researched and are made up of many activities that may be regarded as part of practice. The main elements of professional apprenticeship learning at postgraduate level identified by Macdonald[38] are:

➤ Learning by doing
➤ Experience of seeing patients
➤ Building up personal knowledge and experience
➤ Discussing patients
➤ Managing patients
➤ Having errors corrected
➤ Making teaching points during the course of service
➤ Listening to experts' explanations
➤ 'Picking things up'
➤ Charismatic influences
➤ Learning clinical methods from practice
➤ Being questioned about thought and actions about patients
➤ Teaching by doing
➤ Using knowledge and skill
➤ Bite-size learning from 'bits and pieces'
➤ Retrieving and applying knowledge stored in memory
➤ Learning from supervision
➤ Receiving feedback
➤ Presentation and summarising
➤ Observing experts working
➤ Learning from role models

➤ Learning from teamwork interactions
➤ Hearing consultants thinking aloud
➤ Thinking about practice and patients.

Senior doctors might also recognise much of their learning in some of these elements and will certainly add more – such as conversations with colleagues.

Given such evidence and experience, it is salutary to review the assumptions that seem to be made about doctors' learning when the topic of CPD is discussed.

RIGHT AND WRONG ASSUMPTIONS ABOUT DOCTORS' LEARNING

Conferences and papers about CPD often state the need for doctors to keep up-to-date with a rapidly changing knowledge base and to be accountable to their patients and the public for the standards and modernity of the care they provide. Providing opportunities for learning, or making provision for the 'proper' assessment of learning needs are also frequently mentioned. The literature is overwhelmed with calls for more active approaches to learning based on adult learning theory – although the review of the literature indicates caution on this point. Credit-based schemes of CPD usually specify what types of activity will, or will not, be recognised as being of educational value, implying that some ways of learning are 'better' than others. We have seen that this is not necessarily so.

From such statements, it is possible to infer the assumptions on which they are based. These assumptions often seem quite misconceived. They are shown in the following table.

Wrong assumptions about doctors' learning
➤ Qualified doctors do not continue to learn ➤ Doctors do not assess their learning needs ➤ Doctors ignore service needs in their CPD planning ➤ Doctors are passive learners ➤ There are acceptable and unacceptable ways of learning ➤ Improving practice is not a normal part of professional behaviour ➤ Making doctors learn in approved ways will improve their practice ➤ Doctors do not demonstrate the benefit of CPD undertaken

But does practice not change? Do doctors cope with ever changing circumstances? Brief reflection will suggest that doctors are lifelong learners already and that their practice does change and improve rationally. Any other view is quite unacceptable and flies in the face of reason, evidence and experience. Doctors are not isolated from service planning or from trying to provide the service that their patients and communities want and need. Doctors are at the forefront of the service. It does not take academic research to prove that the negative assumptions and implications about doctors are not only questionable but often absolutely wrong.

Of course, there are doctors who do match up to these negative views – this is almost inevitable in such a large and distributed workforce, but they are the exception not the rule, and they are to be dealt with by systems other than CPD.

The identification of 'approved' methods of learning on the basis of which a doctor can acquire CPD credits is also based on wrong assumptions. We have seen that there is no 'best' method of learning for doctors. The key to effective CPD is in how it is managed not in the method by which it is undertaken.

So, if these assumptions about doctors and continuing learning are wrong, what assumptions are right? The following table answers this question.

Right assumptions about doctors' learning
➤ Are lifelong learners
➤ Do improve and change their practice
➤ Work in a rich learning environment
➤ Have many ways of identifying their learning needs
➤ Have many ways of learning
➤ Are increasingly involved in business planning for the service
➤ Can show the benefit of CPD undertaken

The correctness of these assumptions about doctors' continuing learning is based on the review of the literature on CPD and its effectiveness, and on the research and development work which yielded *The Good CPD Guide*. If we design our educational systems on the basis of the right assumptions, those systems will be effective.

The following pages describe the many ways in which doctors continue to learn and develop. Regulators and professional bodies sometimes do not recognise some of them simply because they are difficult to monitor in terms of hours spent.

It is the credit system as currently implemented that stops effective methods of learning from being recognised.

Nonetheless, these unmonitorable methods are part of the learning environment of every doctor and must be recognised and valued as such within any system of managed CPD because it is not the learning method that determines the effectiveness of the learning, but the stages of needs identification and reinforcement that go before and after it.

If CPD systems are based on the right assumptions, this would lead regulatory bodies to recognise the process of managed CPD for each doctor rather than just recognising the monitorable, quantifiable events of learning that tell only part of the story.

PROFESSIONAL LEARNING METHODS

The many learning methods which doctors use are divided into groups. These are:
➤ Academic activities
➤ Meetings
➤ Learning from colleagues
➤ Learning from practice
➤ Technology-based learning and media
➤ Management and quality processes
➤ Specially arranged events.

ACADEMIC ACTIVITIES

Academic activities are all learning experiences, drawing on and extending doctors' knowledge; involving study, evaluation and discussion of other people's contributions, and the coming together or revision of their own ideas. In many cases, the learning is incidental as well as deliberate. Neither has greater or less value. In short, engagement in academic activities is, by its nature, profoundly educative.

TYPE	METHOD
Academic activities	➤ Writing research papers ➤ Making presentations at conferences and seminars ➤ Refereeing journal articles ➤ Refereeing others' research bids ➤ Medico-legal activity ➤ Reading ➤ Writing and revising service and research protocols ➤ Acting as an external examiner ➤ Teaching

These methods of learning are listed in Appendix 5.

Writing research papers

Of necessity, writing a research paper involves literature review, keeping up to date with research methods, data analysis and reaching conclusions.

Making presentations at conferences and seminars

Preparation for academic presentations also involves mastering the field of knowledge and practice. Needless to say, the conference itself will be educational, but perhaps in unpredictable ways and not linked with a specific need but with the important professional need to keep up-to-date for future unpredictable events.

Refereeing journal articles

Referees are duty bound to be up-to-date and to know the literature and the methods associated with the papers they review. Reading the paper itself can also be an educational event for the reviewer.

Refereeing others' research bids

The need to be up-to-date with the literature and with research methods is required if proper judgments are to be made about others' submissions. Such work can also highlight areas where the reviewer needs to refresh his or her knowledge.

Medico–legal activity

Being an expert witness or otherwise involved in medico-legal cases causes a doctor to think about clinical medicine in ways that are different from that required for daily clinical practice. Lawyers will want to know about detail, derivation, evidence, underlying basic science, basis of clinical judgment, exceptions, related cases and conditions, thinking processes, related clinical skills, health services context and many other aspects of a case. Preparation for medico-legal cases not only reveals areas which require some further personal education, but will also be a learning experience in its own right.

Reading

Literature is at the heart of collected knowledge. It is still at the basis of learning. It is a common stimulus to changing practice. Literature is always available to doctors – whether solicited or not. It is important to have the skills of evaluating the literature read and perhaps discussing it with colleagues. Reading can be opportunistic or well planned; it can be a general or a focused activity. Whichever it is, being aware of its power and the use being made of it will add to its effect and proper application to practice.

Writing and revising service and research protocols

The production of evidence-based protocols for service and research, and protocols for submission for funding, are useful ways of learning and keeping up-to-date, especially when a review of the literature and audit results are involved. For example, a new protocol for the histopathology reporting of colorectal cancer was drawn up by a group of pathologists, based on a review of the literature and results of a region-wide audit. The new protocol provided a useful focus for discussion, and improved and updated practice in this area for pathologists throughout the region.

Grant applications invariably involve a literature review, submissions to ethics committees, maintaining a database and bibliography, perhaps using a computerised system such as Endnote. Having to explain the state of knowledge in a certain field and argue for further research ensures a great deal of learning, thinking and organisation of ideas, as well as helping applicants to hone their written communication skills.

Acting as an external examiner

External examiners are required to be fully informed about the topic they are examining. Reading the thesis, or the examination questions, or contributing to the assessment system, likewise act as a stimulus to the external's own learning.

Teaching

Teaching is a prime example of learning from academic activity. In order to explain something to others, clearly and coherently, teachers have first themselves to understand the way the subject is organised – its key concepts, networks of ideas, methodology, and tests for truth. They must also have detailed, up-to-date theoretical and practical knowledge of particular aspects of it; what is not known has to be researched or experienced before it can be taught. They must also be able to articulate all this, respond to questioning and have their basic understanding interrogated. Furthermore, they need to understand the contribution made by modern teaching technologies and modes of presentation, and be able to use them effectively. The processes involved in carrying out this academic duty are characteristic of what has been termed 'deep' learning: purposeful, self-directed, critical enquiry that is motivated by the desire to know and understand.

MEETINGS

Meetings of various kinds – departmental and inter-departmental, courses, lectures, workshops – are almost daily events in doctors' professional lives, presenting opportunities for different kinds of learning. Meetings have in common that they depend upon processes of communication among groups of people. Often the main purpose of departmental and inter-departmental meetings, for example, is simply to get things done. But, in the process of collective discussion, participants will be learning how the organisation works, how balances of power are struck within it and what reasons lie behind the decisions that are reached. This is important knowledge to have, since everyone concerned works in the organisation and must do so within the framework of the decisions it makes; they need to be able to plan their future courses of action in the light of such knowledge.

Meetings with a more obvious educational purpose can serve to focus a group's attention on a particular topic or issue which, in some cases, the participants might not otherwise give much thought to – a course, lecture or workshop on equal opportunities interviewing procedures, for example. As members of the group begin to confront the possible forms of discrimination enshrined in current practices, they engage in a collective process of analysis and thought. Live discussion of the issues, in particular, encourages shared understandings to develop which may result in individual participants becoming quite committed to views they did even not know they held.

This process may be helped along by breaking down larger discussion groups into clusters of three or four, each with a clear agenda for discussion and certain tasks to accomplish. That way, everyone is encouraged and is able to contribute, and the discussion is focused towards some specific outcome. The small groups may report back their conclusions in plenary session, which also makes discussion in the larger group both feasible and more productive. Apart from what is learned from meetings such as this, group discussion conducted along these lines can have a profound impact on participants' beliefs and attitudes.

Other specific types of meeting are discussed below.

TYPE	METHOD
Meetings	➤ Clinical meetings: departmental and grand rounds ➤ Conferences ➤ Case review ➤ Post-mortems and the clinic-pathological conference (CPC) ➤ Telephone and video conferences

Clinical meetings: departmental and grand rounds

Clinical meetings are designed to be educational by reviewing practice or interesting cases so that all may learn from them. The topics of such meetings are more predictable when they occur in the department rather than on a hospital-wide basis but both will serve an effective educational function by not only being derived from and relevant to practice, but also by offering the opportunity for participation and reflection.

Conferences

Conference attendance is one of the most common formal approaches to learning among doctors and other professionals – and, perhaps, one of the most expensive, but also of key importance to the profession. Sometimes, conferences can be attended for a specific reason, to answer a specific learning need.

On other occasions, and perhaps more commonly, conferences are valuable for general professional learning.

It is commonly believed (although not researched) that the rounded experience of conference attendance includes discussion with peers as much as listening to the programme of presentations, reading the posters or attending workshops. All these aspects of the conference should be recognised and used to their full advantage.

Attendance at conferences often does not produce the specific, goal-directed learning that other events, such as training courses, can achieve. This does not in any way detract from their importance and usefulness. Better understanding, a wider and deeper knowledge base on which to draw in future, new ways of thinking about issues, a better contextual understanding, a feeling of greater confidence, a renewal of energy and all the other positive outcomes of conference attendance will all contribute to better standards of practice.

If attendance at conferences is difficult or impossible, doctors may nowadays experience some of their benefits electronically; accessing the programme and formal papers in a website, or by watching streamed sessions, and 'discussing' the issues involved via forums, or webinars.

Case review meetings

Case reviews can be a most powerful form of learning for all members of the team. Indeed, one of the few circumstances in which multiprofessional learning has been shown to be effective* is in just this environment, where different professionals meet to discuss a real and shared clinical problem in their actual practice. They bring together their knowledge and experience, perhaps reviewing the evidence base for it, and deciding on an approach or a solution. This often involves all members of the team in listening and learning from one another.

Post-mortems and the clinico–pathological conference (CPC)

Discussion between clinician and pathologist can be a valuable learning exercise. The process of arriving at a clinico-pathological correlation can illuminate areas for reflection, improvement in practice and identify learning needs. The post-mortem is a way of looking at clinical outcomes where, for example, the effects of therapy can be demonstrated and the extent of disease elucidated. The clinico-pathological conference is a formalised version of this process.

Telephone and video conferences

Telephone and video conferences are sometimes regarded as best suited to committee work or management discussions. However, both forms of virtual

*See Appendix 1.

meeting are increasingly used in both business and the professions. This is partly due to their decreasing costs as a result of the internet.* Virtual conferences and meetings can be used effectively for teaching and learning. Both telephone and video offer an immediate and interactive form of contact which can reduce the sense of isolation that professionals in remote areas might feel. It can also help people to persist with their own continuing learning or to receive feedback or advice about a particular problem or issue. Telephone teaching and learning can take a number of forms:

➤ One-to-one telephone 'tutorials' with an expert or peer: This is very like an ordinary telephone call or discussion
➤ Small group conference call: This can join up to, perhaps, nine people, all using a domestic telephone,** into a common network, often under the watchful eye of a technical facilitator provided by the telephone company. This call has to be booked in advance with the telephone company. The participants should also prepare for the call by reviewing an agenda or preparatory materials to be discussed in a structured and organised way. There is much room for creativity in such telephone conferences. One of the keys to success is to ensure that there is a 'chairperson' and that contributions are made in an orderly way
➤ Group conference using a telephone with a built-in loudspeaker. This uses a relatively cheap amplifying device around which a group of participants can sit and talk to a remote tutor or expert
➤ Video conferences can be organised using high-end, big screen facilities to link two different centres, or it can be used at the personal level using a lap-top or PC and Skype to link a number of people together. This can be a highly cost-effective and flexible process. But, as with any teaching and learning method, will be best when moderated and prepared for.

Telephone and video conferencing can be used effectively for information transmission, problem-solving, reviewing research, sharing experience and generating ideas.

LEARNING FROM COLLEAGUES

Learning often seems to be something that can only legitimately occur from 'valid sources', from 'experts'. But this view does not reflect the reality of the rich learning environment in which doctors practise and continue to develop: in which they are lifelong learners. The educative effect of senior trainees, of members of the team from other professions (trainees, nurses, pharmacists etc.)

---

*There are many providers of internet services for virtual meetings, Skype being the most widely known.
**This can also be done on the web using services such as Skype.

and even of students, is well-recognised. Learning from members of the team can occur formally, by inviting them to offer presentations or prepare departmental educational meetings, or informally during the course of daily practice and work. Where a specific educational need has been identified, or a team member has indicated an area of knowledge which it would be useful to follow up, then learning from the team becomes an important and valid undertaking.

TYPE	METHOD
Learning from colleagues	➤ Collaborative learning ➤ Consulting other professionals ➤ Joint ward rounds and clinics and professional conversations ➤ Library professionals ➤ Peer review ➤ Peer review: multiprofessional ➤ Peer tutoring ➤ Professional conversations ➤ Visits and travelling clubs ➤ Networking

Collaborative learning

Collaborative learning involves a pair or group of learners distributing the task of learning between them, such that different peers can research and present different aspects of the topic. Alternatively, peers can look at the same aspects of the topic and deepen their understanding by hearing how others approach it. This can be a long-term process or can occur as a strictly time-limited event – for example, of two meetings, the first for distributing the tasks and the second for discussing findings.

Although collaborative learning is the norm for schoolchildren and medical students in problem-based courses, it is not to be found very commonly at postgraduate or continuing education levels. This is, perhaps, not surprising. Arranging to study a topic with another person or with a group of peer learners takes time and organisation. Even although a more thorough acquaintance with the area being studied may well result, the time invested might be seen as out of proportion to the benefit gained. Furthermore, as people develop expertise, their learning needs tend to become more individual – simply because their experience is individual. This is particularly true in the professions. The resultant lack of large areas of shared need for learning might also militate against collaborative learning in medicine. Nonetheless, if the opportunity arises, it is an approach worth trying.

Clinicians' travelling clubs (see below) might be seen as a form of collaborative learning – but the term usually implies something more structured than simply learning together by being together at the same event and discussing it. Groups of doctors who develop guidelines and protocols or who undertake research together might also be seen as collaborative learners benefiting from the community of views and knowledge.

Consulting other professionals

While patients might be getting less reticent about asking for a second opinion, doctors themselves are well used to seeking such opinions both formally and informally. This is a good example of the integration of continuing learning with daily professional practice. It might not be recognised as such by professional bodies, yet it displays all the features of well-constructed learning: an identified need, learning relevant to the need, follow-up, and integration with practice.

Joint ward rounds and clinics, and professional conversations

In some specialties, it is commonplace to conduct ward rounds, and sometimes clinics, with other specialties – for example, with pathologists and pharmacists but also perhaps with community and social services colleagues and with nurses, clinical psychologists, occupational therapists or physiotherapists. A further example is the multidisciplinary team meetings that are widely used in the management of oncology cases. The management of individual cases is discussed and agreed by teams of professionals representing all aspects of care. The professional conversation that occurs about shared cases and the different professional perspectives that are brought to bear in the context of real practice are likely to be powerful sources of learning which, being integrated with practice, can pass without their educational potential and effect ever being accorded their proper importance. Such events are a part of the rich and often unnoticed, learning environment in which health professionals work.

Library professionals (information scientists)

There is much to be learned from professional librarians (now known as information scientists), especially those who work in specialist libraries or, within general libraries, specialise in one's particular academic or professional field. At the least, they can be relied upon to know where to begin looking for any item, however arcane or vague the query. Also, the range of resources available to them is now very wide. Thanks to computerisation of library stocks and search processes, links may be made easily to and items ordered from large, specialist collections, including pictures, newspaper items, audio-visual materials and websites as well as the more standard books and articles. Vast, peer-reviewed collections are always at hand.

These days librarians are trained experts in 'information retrieval' and 'knowledge management'. Part of their job is to teach academics and researchers how to use collections and databases to make their own literature searches, using their computers to explore the catalogues, access lists of specialist journals that regularly publish recent research in the field, and call-up articles and download them. They will also have extensive knowledge of what is available via the internet: those websites dedicated to the specialist field, and the electronic journals and discussion lists that enable researchers to keep up to date with developments.

Librarians often offer dedicated training sessions for those interested in acquiring the skills of information retrieval and management – many are skilled in summarising the literature, for example. Whether learning formally or informally from librarians, they have much to offer which will enhance the effectiveness of CPD.

Peer review

Peer review is useful at all stages of CPD, for identifying learning needs, for learning, and for demonstrating the benefit of learning undertaken. Varieties of peer review are also discussed in Step One.

Peer review is undertaken through internal, external, uni-professional or multiprofessional assessment by peers of the structures, processes and outcomes of the healthcare provided by a unit.

Several specialties now undertake interdepartmental reviews which enable doctors to share and exchange ideas about best clinical or organisational practice. It is perhaps in this type of peer review that effective learning most readily occurs. A measure of the educational effectiveness of such a process was indicated in the area of thoracic medicine[39] where the process involved:

➤ Two reviewers from other departments
➤ Prior collection of basic data on a detailed questionnaire about population, staffing, workload, facilities, training etc.
➤ A two-day visit
➤ Use of published standards and criteria
➤ Production of a detailed report of strengths, weaknesses and recommendations.

On evaluation, 82% of participants felt that they had gained new ideas during the reviews and half the key recommendations for change had been achieved or were imminent after one year. Such peer review thus has a powerful role to play in education and change.

Peer review: multiprofessional

Doctors can learn from other professions, and preparing for and undertaking a formal review of practice which involves other relevant professions can be an informative learning experience. For example, pathology laboratories are subject to regular accreditation and review of all procedures and processes involving all staff, technicians, doctors and administrative and clerical staff. The process of preparing for accreditation involves discussion and review of practice with input on a multiprofessional basis. This process is a learning experience in its own right.

Peer tutoring

Peer tutoring describes much of the continuing learning of a senior doctor. Some of this happens informally, such as when one colleague asks another for an opinion and discusses that opinion, and some is more organised, such as the doctors' travelling clubs (*see* below). Peer tutoring is used at all levels of education and is an approach to learning whereby learners at the same level help each other and learn by teaching and demonstrating practice. It can not only make learning more efficient and pleasurable for those who are taught but can also increase significantly the learning of the tutors.

The benefits of peer tutoring are many. Tutors benefit by:
- Increasing their own sense of personal adequacy
- Using their knowledge and skills to help the development of a colleague
- Reinforcing their own knowledge
- Developing insight into the teaching-learning process.

The person tutored can benefit by:
- Receiving individualised instruction
- Responding to peers
- Comparing personal practice with that of peers
- Receiving the companionship of a colleague in the learning process.

Much of this will happen in any event. However, if peer tutoring is to be a major part of learning, then tutors might need to acquire some skill in the art or think beforehand about:
- How to start the session
- How to give feedback, including praising and correcting (which can be difficult between peers)
- What to do if a session goes badly
- How to vary the content and method of sessions
- How to end a session
- How to keep a record of sessions.

Professional conversations

Contact with other professionals is a powerful stimulus to change. In one study[37], this was a factor in 33% of changes cited. Such professional conversations can take place in many contexts: as part of patient care, at CPD events, during the course of the working day. They may be opportunistic or arranged. They may be casual or focused. It is not surprising that they can be so powerful. Where expertise is based on experience, the vicarious experience of respected fellow professionals can often be as valuable a source of knowledge, as is personal experience. However, judgments must always be made of the interpretation and applicability of all experience, whether of self or others. Being more conscious of such sources of learning may well make those judgments easier to make and more frequently made.

Visits and travelling clubs

Learning from respected colleagues is a fundamental part of professional life. Some specialties have developed this into a well-organised process whereby a group of clinicians will visit another's hospital to attend operations or clinics, to learn about them and to discuss them in detail. Such 'travelling clubs' often take their members abroad, but it is increasingly common for doctors to find that they can learn new techniques and processes from colleagues in neighbouring hospitals or practices. This extension of apprenticeship learning can be a powerful learning experience where colleagues have trust and respect for each other.

Networking

Many CPD activities result in a meeting of professional groups united by a common interest. Such situations provide excellent opportunities for 'networking'. Outside the formal proceedings of the meeting or workshop, old acquaintances can be renewed, new acquaintances formed and matters of mutual professional interest discussed. CPD activity brings new groups and networks into existence. Although networking is not the primary object of the exercise, the benefits are:

➤ News of medical innovation spreading by word of mouth much more rapidly
➤ The development of new collaborative enterprises between individuals, teams or institutions
➤ Doctors are more willing to learn from other doctors than from almost any other source.

LEARNING FROM PRACTICE

It is axiomatic that professionals learn from practice. Just as clinical practice is the basis of postgraduate training, so clinical practice is the basis of continuing expertise once formal training is completed. However, it is not simply the practice itself that ensures continuing learning; it is the thinking about that practice, whether formally or informally. Doctors use many ways of doing this.

TYPE	METHOD
Learning from practice	➤ Diaries ➤ Evidence-based practice ➤ Experiential learning ➤ Mistakes ➤ Opportunistic learning ➤ Portfolio-based learning ➤ Reflective learning

Diaries

Learning diaries are seen in many forms: portfolios and logbooks are the most well-known in medical education. Diaries can be either confidential to the writer or can be shared with peers or an appraiser. Before embarking on it, its purpose and how it is to be filled in and used should be decided. The diary can:

➤ Encourage personal reflection over time
➤ Focus on problems
➤ Record observations and ideas
➤ Provide a record of practice and learning
➤ Be a source for formal discussion with peers or appraiser.

Diaries can range in the degree of their structure. At a minimum, they can simply be filled in at the end of each day with jottings and thoughts. At the other end of the scale, a diary can be highly structured, asking for reflection on specific aspects of practice: communication, clinical skills, record-keeping, team working, etc. Action plans can also be asked for. To be effective, a diary must be filled in regularly and reviewed regularly too. It is likely to be a fruitful exercise as long as the doctor has the time and if the diary is discussed with others. Undertaking the exercise over a defined period with colleagues, perhaps multiprofessionally, might be highly productive.

Evidence-based practice

Evidence-based practice has become something of a watchword in recent years, although exactly what this means in practice is still a matter of debate. So far, it has not generally meant that doctors are referring to the evidence as part of their consultation process but rather that the evidential basis for practice, so far as it exists, is being made more readily available. Thus, guidelines and protocols for practice can be prepared with greater confidence and clinical decisions can be informed more readily by reference to the gathered evidence.

The evidence itself is made available in a variety of forms. There are paper-based 'newsletter' types of missive from professional and government organisations and published reviews from the specialist review centres to which clinicians can readily refer. There are also increasing numbers of electronic information sources that are often updated very frequently. However, not all of these will live up to the standards of the Cochrane-type databases, and care should be exercised in their use. The Cochrane Database of Systematic Reviews (CDSR) and the York Database of Abstracts of Reviews of Effectiveness (DARE), the Cochrane Controlled Trials Register and the Cochrane Review methodology database are all well-respected.

Other developments, such as the OVID Core Collection, provide hypertext links from references in Medline to the original article in electronic form that can then be printed out. The plethora of national and international evidence sources has meant that hospitals are considering setting up their own internal intranet sources, often drawing on the wider web-based sources. Cochrane databases made available in the labour ward are an example of this. It requires considerable technical support to set up and maintain such a system. Clinicians should make sure that they have input into the design stage so that appropriate ease of access is made more likely. As a source of information and evidence, reference to such databases and reviews as are available is undoubtedly a potentially useful learning method that can be linked directly to practice.

Experiential learning

Learning from experience includes learning from mistakes (*see* below), learning from an ever-increasing portfolio of patients seen and their outcomes, and learning from the daily events of clinical work such as ward rounds. It is the most important way in which all professionals continue to learn. Educationalists offer a variety of ways of improving on this professionally integrated and unavoidable 'situated learning' and according to the advice offered; tend to call it different things: reflective learning (*see* below) is one such approach to developing what professionals do already. Experiential learning is another. Some would say that these two are much the same, and this would seem to be the case if we look at one of the most significant theorists in the field[40] who, in the 1970s, identified a learning cycle made up of:

➤ Concrete experience
➤ Observation and reflection
➤ Formation of abstract concepts and generalisations
➤ Testing implications of the concepts in new situations.

This seems to describe what doctors do. They learn from their experience and apply what they have learned to their future practice. It is undoubtedly the case that this method of professional learning could be made more explicit and conscious and so could benefit learning in practice even more. Given that educationalists offer a wide variety of potential ways of doing this (many of which remain untested), it might be best for the individual clinician to decide which of these to choose for personal use. Many of the learning methods described in this section apply – for example, portfolio-based learning, case review, audit, peer learning and many others.

Mistakes

When a clinical mistake has been made, this can be a trigger for individual reflection and identification of learning needs, as well as organisational review. An analysis of the reason for the mistake must be made. For example, was the mistake due to:

➤ Lack of knowledge?
➤ Overwork and stress?

➤ Inadequate protocols or guidance?
➤ Contextual issues?

Appropriate learning can then be planned. Such learning in practice is likely to be powerful in affecting future practice.

Opportunistic learning

Many of the learning methods cited in this section show the inevitable integration of learning and practice - to practise medicine is to learn more about it. This is true at postgraduate level as well as for the established doctor. Opportunistic learning occurs as a result of an unusual or interesting incident or event that is immediately followed up. For example, a patient may present with or raise an unfamiliar aspect of disease or its consequences, or a colleague might mention a new development. A chance meeting with an expert, academic or other colleague can result in following up a known learning need or simply learning something new. Such events are thus a trigger to learning in many ways and are not to be underestimated in their importance simply because they are entirely unplanned and unpredictable. They are often more memorable just for that.

Portfolio-based learning

Learning portfolios are a developing but largely unproven approach to learning in medicine. The method is described in Step One of this Guide and is often used to show that learning has occurred rather than as a learning method *per se*. However, ways of using portfolios for learning have also been described. This involves the learner in actively reflecting on the contents of the portfolio and drawing out what has been learned. This is best done with a trainer or colleague, who can listen, challenge statements, clarify, summarise and reflect back to the learner what has been said.

Reflective learning

For many years, reflection on experience has been recognised as a centrally important learning method within continuing education in all the professions. This recognition arose out of certain underlying beliefs about the nature of adult learning in general: that adults' own needs should be met through education that is lifelong, engages with and progressively builds on their experience; and that the aim of adult education is to foster self-directed, empowered adults who are able to reflect critically on their professional and personal life and on the society in which they live and work.[41,42] Yet enduring criticisms of continuing education provision suggest that these principles have not been applied successfully in practice. Courses are often seen as largely irrelevant to the participants' professional and practical needs, as too theoretical and too didactic. Schön has argued that this is because in all professions, 'scientific' (theoretical) knowledge has been valued most highly, so that relationships between theoretical knowledge and practice are not well understood while practical professional knowledge and skill are persistently undervalued.

Schön's approach to resolving this 'rigor or relevance' dilemma involves uncovering the knowledge that he regards as inherent in skilful performance – the sequence of procedures, clues observed, rules followed and the values, strategies and assumptions that make up 'theories of action' – through processes of 'reflection-in-action' and 'reflection-on-action'. Essentially, these are cognitive processes that deal critically with previous activity and thought. A range of techniques for encouraging such reflection has been developed subsequently, along with other strategies for ensuring that continuing education fosters practical competence. In medicine these include:

➤ Stimulated recall (sometimes based on video recordings)[43]
➤ Task analysis[44]
➤ The Delphi technique
➤ Behavioural event interview[45]
➤ And critical incident surveys.

Each aims to explore and make explicit doctors' own thought processes or experiences and perceptions of events. Some less formal ways of stimulating reflection on experience, referred to elsewhere in this Guide, include keeping a diary, taking a sabbatical, being attached or seconded to other hospitals, and visiting colleagues overseas. However, an interest in method and technique should not blind us to Schön's penetrating analysis of the underlying importance of the cultural history of the professions (their structures, assumptions and power relations) as they affect both the learning needs of individual practitioners and the kind of continuing education provision that is actually offered. The analysis suggests that a thorough-going overhaul of provision must wait upon some radical re-conceptualisation within and of the professions themselves. It is hoped *The Good CPD Guide* might contribute to this process within.

TECHNOLOGY-BASED LEARNING AND MEDIA

Technology is increasingly part of both practice and learning.

TYPE	METHOD
Technology-based learning and media	➤ Audio-visual ➤ Communication and information technologies ➤ Computer support systems ➤ Distance learning/blended learning ➤ Mass media and open sources ➤ Simulations ➤ Live interactive events ➤ Video review of performance ➤ Social media for learning

Audio-visual

Audio-visual modes of learning are now commonplace in most forms of education and training. Within the highly visual subject of medicine, doctors will be most familiar with learning from specially-made videos. For example, an entire surgical procedure can be recorded, as performed by an expert, and viewed subsequently by large numbers of other experts and doctors in training. Or the video may be edited, with particularly interesting passages in the operation highlighted and shown close-up or from angles that only the camera can access. Such presentations can be copied or distributed quite cheaply, for use by individual viewers who are then in control; they may replay sections of the recording for particularly close inspection.

The fundamentally important process of diagnosis also depends upon close observation. In neurology, for example, the subject's physical appearance, movements and gait will be highly suggestive. Here, short videos may be used to stimulate discussion among an audience. Videoconferencing allows doctors to discuss a case while simultaneously presenting visual evidence, in real time across vast distances. And live video links, through telemedicine (*see* below), are increasingly being used to aid diagnosis 'in the field', enabling visual as well as aural communication between paramedics at the scene of an accident or GPs in remote locations and specialists back in the hospital.

Sound-only media should not be forgotten. Talks by specialists and discussion between them may be presented in sound alone, with the absence of rich visual images, actually aiding concentration. As a cheap, highly portable and flexible medium, hand-held recording devices also enable the 'authentic' voice of the patient to be heard, in naturalistic settings such as home or surgery. Moreover, audio recording used in combination with vision (pictures, diagrams, specimens, slides, tables of statistics) – in, for example webinars (web-based seminars) or interactive tutorials – is still a powerful learning medium; people can be 'talked through', prompted and guided as they practise a manual skill, find the correct column in a table or examine particular features of a specimen, replaying parts of the soundtrack whenever they need to. Although most often used in distance learning, such techniques can be widely effective, especially towards scrutinising objects with great care and developing skills involving hand-eye co-ordination.

Podcasts and videocasts are pre-recorded audio and/or video tracks which can be downloaded to a computer or a portable device for viewing or listening. While many podcasts are entertainment, several institutions are choosing to deliver their content in this form, for example by making it available through iTunes U.*

---

*You will need to download the software. If you are in the UK, go to www.apple.com/uk/itunes/affiliates/download/?id=403519008

Communication and information technologies

There are many new technologies that have rapidly become part of our everyday lives. These, however, can be valuable tools for undertaking a variety of learning activities.

First are those tools that aid collaborative learning – in which people work together, discuss their ideas and share information. Particularly important here are email, list-serves, web-based groups, discussion forums and the networked systems of communication (computer and videoconferencing). Email enables one-to-one or one-to-many communication across the world.

E-conferencing is an extension of this principle. Using dedicated websites or software, a group of people can collaborate, share and discuss. A topic of discussion is begun (perhaps by a teacher or conference moderator) and anyone in the group can send a message to it, which everyone else can read and anyone may reply to. Some participants perhaps log on every day, replying to messages quite frequently; some may do so only once a week, reading through all the messages that have been posted in the meantime before responding to one or more of them – this is an asynchronous, text-based mode of communication. These conferences can also be conducted as webinars, where all participants log on at the same time and are present as they would be in a seminar or tutorial.

Video can also be part of these conferences and sophisticated techniques are possible, such as use of computer-generated graphics and split-screen presentations, which require technical skill and resources. Videoconferencing clearly has its advantages, particularly in those highly visual subjects such as medicine, but it requires people (possibly located in different time zones) to be present at a predetermined time and place. It also requires far greater investment in equipment and technical support.

Second is e-learning: those technologies that assist more independent or self-directed learning and tend to favour knowledge acquisition, which are mostly delivered via the internet. These multimedia resources are often produced by experts or commercial companies, and are interactive. They can be expensive to make and to use. Self-assessment questions and other devices such as notebook and copy facilities may be present, again depending on whether the resource has a predominant teaching/learning or reference function. Although it appears difficult to verify the accuracy and value of a resource, sites that are not to be trusted or are inaccurate will quickly receive negative feedback. Reading reviews of sites before embarking on a programme of learning, or only using those that are peer-reviewed, will weed out those which are not a valuable resource.

Most recently, using platforms such as Moodle, educational institutions are setting up their own websites to enable on-line learning in the 'virtual classroom'. That is, the tools for both collaborative and independent forms of learning are being brought together in the same 'place'. In principle, having entered the site, students may:

➤ Take part in a computer conference
➤ Search a course text or database
➤ Watch a video
➤ Access other, recommended websites
➤ Download a diagram to paste into another document
➤ Send a completed assignment to their tutor (who will mark and return it electronically)
➤ Send an e-mail to a collaborator in project work
➤ Have a chat with friends in the 'cyber-cafe'.

Planning and preparation are essential to these real-time interactions.

Computer support systems

Computer support systems are not primarily intended as a method of learning but are rather intended to offer an information base and guidelines for active decisions made in the course of patient care. Many computerised patient record systems already offer this facility. Separate systems can offer recommendations on prescribing and management issues for the most frequently seen clinical conditions and can issue reminders and predict doses of prescribed drugs, as well as alerts to drug interactions, allergies and contraindications.

Other systems are available, such as that for the management of cardiovascular risk factors. There is some evidence that computer support systems influence prescribing behaviour.[46] To that extent, they are a learning method.

Distance learning/blended learning

Distance and blended learning are now becoming more common in medical education at all levels. Typically, distance learners are adults who study part-time from home, the workplace or a local centre. They are separated in time and space from the teaching institution, teachers and other learners. Some face-to-face tuition and other learning experiences should be available within the blend, but distance learners mainly study independently from specially prepared text and audio-visual material or through computer-based learning methods.

Distance learning (or self-instructional) materials are designed with these learners' needs in mind:

➤ In recognition of the absence of a teacher on hand, explanations are clear and full, examples are provided, and learners are addressed in an informal, friendly tone
➤ Because distance learners receive relatively little face-to-face feedback, self-assessment items are usually included and assignments are returned quickly by the learner's tutor, along with written comments
➤ It is assumed that the time available for study is limited, so a reasonable workload is inbuilt and the pace of study is carefully regulated

➤ Because study periods are likely to be short or interrupted, care is taken to provide easy access to the material (which may be presented in blocks or as modules) as well as frequent summary of contents
➤ As far as possible, the material is designed to be used flexibly; by a wide range of people, at the learners' own pace and in their own place of study.

Distance learning is, therefore, a particularly appropriate mode in any professional continuing education context. The only proviso here is that there must be a relatively large number of people who will study any one distance learning course for it to be cost-effective.

Mass media and open sources

The mass media of broadcast television and radio, newspapers and magazines are more often used to keep the general public informed about medical matters than to provide information or a forum for doctors themselves. The occasional features are most instructive as a measure of shifting opinion and perceptions of the professions within popular culture.

Equally revealing in this respect is the way hospital life is represented in story, drama and soap opera. But these representations are also powerful perception-formers. Just as patients may require reassurance about sensational news stories concerning the effects of drugs, or of particular foodstuffs on people's health, so certain ideas or prejudices picked up from fictional accounts may need to be addressed. For this reason, it is well worth doctors being aware of what is going on in the mass media and trying to assess its meaning and significance as a deliberate educational activity.

Open sources, such as the myriad public and commercial health advice sites, and others such as Wikipedia, have made the internet the first port-of-call for the majority of the public, and for some students and professionals too. These are useful but peer review of the content must always be considered.

Simulations

Medical education is no stranger to simulations in the form of skills laboratories for clinical examination and communication, of actors, simulated patients, physical simulations for surgical skills, mannequins for examination skills etc. In general practice, simulated surgeries are well known for the purposes of learning and assessment. Simulations offer varying degrees of reality replication. Paper-and-pencil or computer-based patient management problems, for example, are a representation of the clinical decision-making process which is abstracted rather than offering high fidelity. On the other hand, for a long time, it has been difficult to differentiate some standardised patients from the real thing.[47] Increasingly, simulations are relying on computer technology – the virtual microscope and virtual brain being good examples. Simulations can be used to help people learn anything from a specific skill, to the whole integrated process of diagnosis and patient management. There is much research to support their use and testify to their effectiveness.[48]

Live interactive events

New procedures pioneered in a particular place may be relayed directly to other sites via live feed, with an audio link also enabling viewers to question surgeons as they work. These methods of learning from expert performance may actually be preferred to presence in the operating theatre, which provides a more limited view for only a few, especially when participants can raise questions and discuss the procedure as it progresses.

Telemedicine is usually taken to mean the use of live television links to facilitate patient care by, for example, linking a GP surgery with a department of accident and emergency so that the hospital consultant's opinion can be sought about patients attending the surgery during their actual consultation. This, of course, can be a learning experience in its own right for the doctor seeking the second opinion. Teleradiology, telepathology and teleconsulting are already well-established on both sides of the Atlantic. However, more deliberate educational uses are being, and can be, made of such links, as the Royal College of Surgeons of England live-links programme for teaching minimal access surgery has demonstrated. Such a system links operating theatres and a 'classroom', perhaps backed up with simulations. A group of learners is in the classroom and watches the operation performed by the surgeon at the remote site. Questions to the operating surgeon are allowed so that discussion of the operation as it proceeds is offered. The learners can have simulated practice of the focal techniques before, during or after the operation.

Video review of performance

Video recording activities is a powerful way to review one's own performance, to learn and to show that improvement has occurred. Any behaviour may be videoed, and examples include practical skills such as joint injection and management skills such as appraisal. The most common application of video assessment is probably the review of the communication skills used in a patient encounter; the consultation. There are three main stages to using video assessment:

➤ Producing a recording with high-quality image and sound, after obtaining patient consent
➤ Reviewing the recording, individually or with others
➤ Documenting the learning and incorporating it into future behaviour.

Written patient consent is necessary before and after the recording. There must also be a procedure for storing and destroying or recording over saved videos.

Video review of performance has several advantages. It:
➤ Examines what you do rather than what you think you do
➤ Acknowledges good behaviour
➤ Provides opportunity to enhance skills
➤ Provides peer insights
➤ Suggests new strategies.

However, it also has disadvantages that include:
➤ Initial equipment cost
➤ Time-consuming
➤ Anxiety/vulnerability
➤ Opportunity for destructive criticism.

Social media for learning

Social media is a conversation that takes place online. Those engaged in learning can engage with others of like mind, and discuss, collaborate and learn, in both a formal and informal setting. Sites such as LinkedIn provide professional links and recommendations, whereas Twitter and Facebook have created a revolution of connectivity and contact.

Patients and the public increasingly expect a professional presence on Twitter and Facebook; active Twitter users such as NHS Choices* have thousands of followers. Twitter is a mine of real-time information, often beating the BBC news website for breaking news, but it is unclear at this stage whether micro-blogging will play a role in professional collaboration.

Professional blogs, however, are a very useful way of learning. Experts can write detailed (and lengthy) posts about their interests, experiences and thoughts, which can be read by anyone who shares those particular interests.

There are obvious limitations. Social media can be accessed by anyone, anywhere, and therefore issues of patient confidentiality must be respected. Social media cannot replace the valuable experience of professionals discussing their craft in person, but by increasing the potential audience, the benefits are increased. Online discussion and collaboration must complement and not replace face-to-face interaction.

Technology is increasingly part of both practice and learning. As a source of information or a means of storing it, there is much to be learned from using technologies.

MANAGEMENT AND QUALITY PROCESSES

The ever-increasing range of management and quality processes now include those that encompass an account of continuing education, such as revalidation.

*www.nhs.uk/Pages/HomePage.aspx

TYPE	METHOD
Management and quality processes	➤ Accreditation: hospital ➤ Audit ➤ Inspection visits ➤ Quality assessment schemes ➤ Revalidation

Accreditation: hospital

Accreditation of hospitals or of their individual departments depends upon their ability to demonstrate that the hospital or department complies with a set of standards. These standards may be generated by the organisation itself or may be external. Some accreditation schemes depend on generating adherence to standards more related to general management than to clinical practice. More clinically orientated systems depend upon a hospital or a department having the ability to deliver care according to accepted protocols or guidelines such as those produced by the medical Royal Colleges or the specialist societies in the UK. For doctors in an individual department, the process of undergoing accreditation provides the opportunity to become thoroughly familiar with the standards themselves, the guidelines and protocols upon which they may be based and the underlying rationale for those guidelines. There is also a need to become thoroughly familiar with the roles and responsibilities of other staff working in the department. Finally, there are less easily defined beneficial learning experiences involved: the cooperation needed within a department to achieve demanding standards depends upon those involved in leading the process having high levels of team-building and change management skills.

Audit

Audit is designed to change practice or to confirm that practice is acceptable. However, since its inception, its educational potential has been analysed[49] as having the following components:
➤ It promotes group working, modifying attitudes and approaches to clinical problems; people learning to work together more effectively
➤ It enhances critical approaches and gives a rational basis to change
➤ It encourages learning about new techniques and treatments
➤ By describing required standards of practice, it gives guidance as to what is expected.

Inspection visits

Inspection is a fundamental process in many aspects of medicine, whether it is inspection of education, or inspection of clinical units and clinical practice for purposes of recognition or accreditation. This form of the 'clinical method' is well-respected and is a powerful learning experience both for those inspected and those who inspect. But the specific lessons are rarely recorded as such. Neither is all the work that underpins such visits on both sides. Specific recording of what has been learned and how it was learned would reveal another rich seam in the integrated learning that underpins professional life.

Quality assessment schemes

Quality assessment schemes are most prevalent and established in the laboratory specialties. However, other clinical specialties might look at these and decide whether or not something similar could be of value to them. For example, diagnostic histopathology external quality assessment (EQA) schemes in the UK and elsewhere involve the circulation of 'test' material to participants, usually consisting of histological sections and appropriate clinical information. Diagnoses and comments are returned to the organiser of the scheme and reports relating to individual performance are returned to the participants. The educational component of EQA relates to the intrinsic learning value of looking at the cases and also to the feedback that is provided for each participant.

Revalidation

Revalidation of a doctor's registration is a process which, in general, includes:

> '… appraisal and assessment, standards that doctors will need to meet in order to revalidate, and colleague and patient feedback questionnaires'*

Revalidation is inextricably linked to education: the reflection on practice that it entails will be a process of learning in its own right and will stimulate further personal and organisational development.

> Revalidation is a formal system for ensuring that doctors remain fit for practice. It is a positive affirmation that doctors are safe and keeping up-to-date, rather than just an absence of concerns**

SPECIALLY ARRANGED EVENTS

As well as the learning opportunities that present themselves during the course of the working week, or are provided by others in the form of conferences and meetings, clinicians also have the opportunity to arrange special educational events for themselves. These are sometimes quite elaborate and can require considerable planning.

*General Medical Council. www.gmc-uk.org/doctors/7330.asp
**Faculty of Forensic and Legal Medicine. http://fflm.ac.uk/education/revalidation/

TYPE	METHOD
Specially arranged events	➤ Attachments and secondments ➤ Sabbaticals

Attachments and secondments

Working in another hospital, whether in the home country or overseas, is an excellent opportunity for learning. Free from anxiety about future employment, doctors on attachment or secondment are immersed in the way of life of a different institution, a different form of departmental organisation and perhaps of clinical approach and method, for an appreciable period. In some cases, for example, secondment from a district general hospital to a more specialised institution, or a period spent in research rather than clinical practice, doctors may be able to try out new techniques and develop new skills, thus deepening and/or broadening their knowledge and experience.

In any case, comparison between previous and current experience and debate among new colleagues can be invigorating, as well as instructive. The break from day-to-day routine tends to 'distance' doctors from their previous assumptions, with the new environment both enabling and stimulating critical reflection and reassessment of their practices (*see* 'Reflective Learning', above). This is perhaps particularly true of attachments or secondments overseas, when the culture within which medicine is practised is very different. Wider exposure to Asian medical philosophy, for instance, has no doubt increased acceptance by western doctors of alternative, more holistic, practices, including a role for acupuncture, and greater attention to diet and relaxation. Doctors who regularly work among minority ethnic groups may find a visit to the country of origin of immediate practical benefit, both to themselves and their patients.

But wherever the attachment, such a mind-broadening experience is invariably educative in itself.

Sabbaticals

A sabbatical is an extended period of leave for travel and study, often a year, which is granted at intervals during a doctor's career. As such, the institution offers long-term employees the chance to drop the day-to-day habits and concerns of the job, and instead become fully immersed in activities that have an updating and refreshing function or that extend the doctor's interests and skills, in breadth or depth. A long period of leave provides the time to undertake a substantial research or writing project, to extend the horizons by visiting colleagues in other hospitals, community centres and abroad, to attend conferences and meetings, to catch-up with developments in areas adjacent to the job or to make a long-term investment in acquiring a new clinical, educational or managerial skill. Clearly, all these activities involve a good deal of learning of various kinds.

However, what this list of possibilities reveals is the wide range of options open to the doctor about to take a sabbatical, and it highlights certain dangers.

First, there is a danger that it will take far more time than anticipated for the doctor to become really involved in a project of any kind. Also, all those activities listed would require some organisation well in advance. That means deciding what exactly will be attempted, at least during the first few months of leave, and then making the necessary arrangements – especially if the plan involves other people's time, travel, ordering equipment and study material or booking accommodation. Obviously, these plans should be realistic rather than over-ambitious. It is a good idea to talk them through with colleagues, especially those who have taken a sabbatical before, not only because they may have sound advice and good ideas to offer but also because this gives the project an air of reality; from the start there is the sense that certain things are expected and must be accomplished.

Second, once started on the sabbatical, there is the danger of loss of momentum. The time may seem to stretch ahead so that there is no real urgency about anything. This feeling is, of course, one of the joys of a sabbatical but it needs to be kept within bounds. It helps to set targets for the completion of short projects or for stages in the progress of a longer one. The targets may be missed, but at least they will be known to have been missed and can be redrawn.

And finally, a commitment at the outset to sharing the results of the sabbatical with colleagues back in the hospital or practice will have a double function. It provides an incentive to actually complete the projects undertaken and an opportunity for further learning in discussion with others; and it gives the institution some return on its 'investment' in the sabbatical.

STEP FOUR: USE THE LEARNING AND SHOW ITS EFFECT

The Good CPD Guide shows that to be effective, CPD must be used and followed up in some way. Such follow-up has three main purposes:
➤ It reinforces the learning in the practice context
➤ It allows for dissemination of the learning to others
➤ It allows the overall effectiveness of the CPD to be judged.

STEP	METHOD	EFFECT

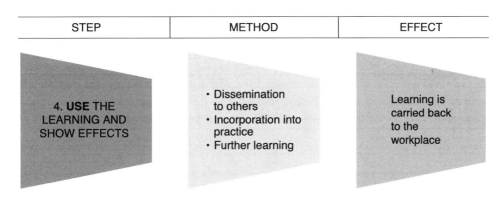

4. USE THE LEARNING AND SHOW EFFECTS

- Dissemination to others
- Incorporation into practice
- Further learning

Learning is carried back to the workplace

REINFORCING LEARNING

While educationalists constantly develop new theories and methods of teaching and learning, the positive effects of reinforcing learning is one accepted feature of education and training that has not changed for many decades. Neither is it likely to. In medical education, also, it is one of the few features of CPD, along with purpose and relevance that has been shown to be important in generating positive outcomes.[50]

Reinforcement of learning can take very many forms – repeating the learning, revisiting it, using it, applying it, explaining it, re-evaluating it, teaching it to others, summarising it, and so on. If the reinforcement occurs in the place where the learning has to be applied, then so much the better.

Doctors have very many ways of reinforcing the learning gained through CPD. In this section, the most common of these are described.

DISSEMINATING THE CPD LOCALLY

In any department or practice, it is clearly desirable that new information and skills should be disseminated as widely as possible. If a doctor who has been away on a CPD event plans to undertake an activity to spread the learning to colleagues, this has self-evident value in providing reinforcement of the learning, as well as ensuring that it is brought back to the team and the practice environment, increasing its likelihood of being used.

MEASURING THE EFFECTIVENESS OF CPD: THE CHALLENGES

Those who undertake CPD have a responsibility to show that it has been of benefit. However, there are major difficulties in undertaking outcome research in education under any circumstances. Educational events are rarely isolated activities, specific outcomes are often difficult to identify, and even more difficult to measure.

> There are often many intervening or contaminating variables between the educational event and the outcome, which make it impossible to attribute cause and effect.

In medicine, there are myriad uncontrolled, and unknown, variables associated with the characteristics and circumstances of doctors, patients and their relationships. These factors all make it inappropriate to aspire to demonstrate a measurable, causal relationship between CPD and a specific outcome in other than a few specific circumstances. The following table summarises the problem:

Table 1: Challenges in a relationship between CPD and outcomes

Aspects	Intervening variables	Difficulties posed
Learners	➤ Individual differences in attitudes, needs, experience, expectations, preferred learning activities. ➤ Differences in characteristics of those affected by learners' behaviours.	➤ How can these differences be isolated, described and classified? ➤ What are the influences of differences on the rest of the process? ➤ How can these be evaluated?
CPD activity	➤ Varieties in quality and content of educational provision. ➤ Varieties in the extent to which the needs of learners and client groups are addressed.	➤ How should CPD activities be evaluated? ➤ How can programmes be described and compared?
Changes in learners	➤ Changes achieved may or may not be those relating to identified needs of learners and/or client groups. But might be useful, nonetheless.	➤ What should be evaluated when? ➤ What methods of evaluation should be used?

Changes in professional practice	➤ Changes achieved might or might not be those which had been planned/anticipated. ➤ Varieties in magnitude and scope of changes.	➤ Which measuring tools are the most appropriate?
Changes in outcomes of practice or in patient attributes	➤ Varieties in the timing of the emergence of changes and of their persistence. ➤ Varieties of patient circumstance. ➤ The outcome might be that the doctor's current practice is confirmed as best practice; so no change is required.	➤ Should behaviour and outcomes be compared with absolute criteria or evaluated in terms of personal advance? ➤ Are there unexpected outcomes? ➤ What is the appropriate timescale for measurement? ➤ How is 'no change' to be recorded as an important outcome?

What, then, is to be done? The capacity to know that a subject has been learned, and to demonstrate that, is part of the essential characteristics of professional continuing, self-directed learning. The solution to the challenge of doing this is to adopt methods that are, themselves, characteristic of professional behaviour, rather than adopting an evidence-based 'research model', unless that is entirely appropriate.

> The outcomes of continuing professional development are difficult to measure in a meaningful way. A new approach to proof of effect is required, which looks at the professional process rather than correlations of unknown value or generalisability.

This section describes many such ways that doctors have of completing the CPD cycle by using the CPD they have undertaken. Those ways have the dual advantage of also being methods of reinforcement and dissemination of the learning. These are summarised in Appendix 6.

It is useful at this stage to repeat Step 4 (*see* page 69).

WHO BENEFITS FROM CPD?

The benefits of showing that CPD was worthwhile may accrue to a wide range of different individuals, groups and institutions. At one level, the promotion through CPD of an effective approach to the prevention or treatment of illness may be of great benefit to the Treasury. At a more local level, hospital trusts, departments, primary care groups and practices clearly have an interest in maintaining the highest possible standards of service. Such standards are an appropriate aspiration for their own sake, but they are also of major importance in risk management.

At the other end of the scale, a single episode of CPD may be of immediate benefit only in the personal development of an individual practitioner. But this will affect many patients. Departments, hospital trusts, practices and ultimately the whole NHS will rely on such personal development to meet the challenges of the future. Finally, it is important to stress that the driving force behind the whole of CPD is the desire to provide high-quality medical services to patients, and that patients are the ultimate beneficiaries of good CPD.

TYPES OF CHANGE RESULTING FROM CPD: HOW CAN THEY BE APPRECIATED?

It is conventional to regard a change in practice as the normal benefit from CPD activity. In many cases, this is appropriate. For example, where an individual has undertaken training in a new surgical technique, the hospital trust and department will clearly expect to be able to provide this new service for their patients and to see it performed effectively and safely. But …

A major element of many CPD activities is concerned with confirming that an individual's current clinical practice is of a high standard. It follows that a CPD activity may not lead to any change in clinical practice and that this is a perfectly satisfactory outcome.

This is so, not least because patients may receive exactly the same treatment before and after their doctor has undertaken a CPD activity, and the only change may be the doctor's heightened confidence that his or her own clinical practice really does conform to contemporary best practice.

Such personal concern to ensure that one's own practice meets high standards lies at the heart of a professional commitment. The same applies to any service for which a doctor is responsible, even though that doctor may not deliver all the clinical services personally.

For appropriately reflective practitioners, much of their personal reading time and time spent attending meetings will be accompanied by a continuous internal process of checking that what they are reading or hearing fits with their own practice. Such a process is internal and clearly not amenable to any external system of scoring or counting. In this respect, it does not differ from many other aspects of professional practice.

Conscientious professionals need to know that what they are doing is based on good evidence. In many areas of practice the evidence is incomplete or uncertain and, in such areas, professionals need to know that their practice accords with that of reputable colleagues. The opportunity to undertake appropriate CPD fulfils these needs. Moves to promote and foster a strong professional culture, where good medical practice is perceived as a central personal duty, will strengthen the determination of individual clinicians to relate all their learning back to their individual practice. Such a strong professional culture is the cornerstone of high quality practice.

SHOWING THE EFFECTIVENESS OF CPD

One of the characteristics which we notice in departments that are recognised to be excellent is that the doctors (and other staff) in the department are well-informed, skilful in their clinical, teaching and managerial activities and enthusiastic about their work. They keep up-to-date. These effects of continuing learning are hard to measure directly but they might be the most important outcome of CPD.

The positive effects of CPD may be at a variety of different levels: personal, departmental, institutional, in terms of the service, the care of patients, costs, techniques, skills, attitudes. A measure directed at identifying short-term observable change might not be appropriate. Long-term changes and changes simply in confidence might be more appropriate.

> In the end, nothing specifically measurable might be found – but professional judgment of unmeasurable qualities can be as valuable and valid as quantitative data that can only measure the measurable and thereby often miss the significant factors.

Given this, it is important to be aware of the methods of using the CPD undertaken and so reinforcing and disseminating the new learning and demonstrating that its benefits are integrated with the professional practice of doctors. Thus, formal methods of assessment are not included in *The Good CPD Guide* – and are often inappropriate for all these reasons.

The ultimate aim of CPD is that patients may be able to go to practices and hospital departments where the staff they meet are knowledgeable, skilled and enthusiastic. In such circumstances, the standard of treatment the patient receives is inevitably high, given that the organisation can support it. It is often easier to appreciate the global benefits of CPD in this sort of context, rather than attempting to reduce the benefits to component parts. It has proved impossible to identify any established methodology capable of producing quantitative information on the global benefits of CPD activity. However …

> Following the effective CPD cycle, described here, will ensure that the new learning is used. Showing how this was done should be allowed in any way appropriate to the CPD undertaken.

The use made of the new learning might be in any domain and manner. Showing effect should be reviewed periodically but the methods of demonstrating effect must be flexible enough to encompass the wide variety of outcome. By using some of the approaches set out below, it may be possible to refine the process of review and achieve greater understanding.

METHODS OF USING CPD AND SHOWING ITS EFFECTS

A variety of methods of following up CPD by using the learning, for reinforcement, dissemination and to show its effectiveness are described below. They are methods that are formal and informal, institutional and personal. Most serve a variety of purposes. They are not, therefore, amenable to categorisation according to their main use. Accordingly, they are presented in alphabetical order after the following table which indicates the usefulness of each approach discussed.

We asked doctors how they followed up their CPD and judged that it had had an effect. Their answers, and the literature review, form the basis of the following table. It does not contain direct measurement of patient characteristics or changes, for the reasons discussed above.

Table 2: Methods of following up CPD and showing its effectiveness

Method	Main function			
	Use		To show effectiveness	
	Reinforcement of learning	Dissemination of learning	For the organisation	For the doctor
Accreditation/ certification of the individual				✔
Accreditation of services			✔	✔
Appraisal			✔	✔
Assessment of learning			✔	✔
Assessment results of trainees			✔	✔
Audit	✔	✔	✔	✔

Method	Reinforcement of learning	Dissemination of learning	For the organisation	For the doctor
Changes in person specification			✔	✔
Changing practice	✔	✔	✔	✔
Clinical effectiveness			✔	✔
CPD credit points				?
Collaborative assessment	✔	✔	✔	
Confidence levels				✔
Corporate image			✔	
Decreasing professional isolation				✔
'Don't know' factor			✔	✔
Educational culture			✔	
Educational records and log-books				?
Effects on the team			✔	✔
Enhancing practice	✔		✔	✔
Learning diaries	✔			✔
Learning portfolios	✔			✔
New services	✔	✔	✔	✔
Obsolete and inappropriate practice	✔	✔	✔	✔
Peer review of the medical team			✔	✔
Personal invigoration				✔
Protection from successful litigation			✔	✔

continued

Method	Reinforcement of learning	Dissemination of learning	For the organisation	For the doctor
Recruitment of medical staff			✔	
Reduction in burnout and early retirement			✔	✔
Referrals to the doctor			✔	✔
Remunerative benefit				✔
Reporting back to colleagues	✔	✔	✔	✔
Reputation as a trainer			✔	✔
Research	✔	✔	✔	✔
Risk management	✔		✔	
Self-assessment	✔			✔
Time-efficient working			✔	✔
Video assessment	✔	✔		✔
Written reports	✔	✔		✔

THE METHODS

Accreditation/certification of the individual

The process of certification or accreditation of individual specialists self-evidently depends upon demonstration that the specialist has met certain predetermined educational standards. The process may involve a small area of an individual's practice, such as certification of the skills required for resuscitation provided by the ATLS (Advanced Trauma Life Support) and ACLS (Advanced Cardiac Life Support) courses of the Resuscitation Council. Alternatively, it may extend across an individual's entire practice as, for example, will be the case in revalidation.

Re-certification and re-accreditation processes generally depend upon demonstration that an individual has taken part in appropriate educational processes rather than on formal assessment of what they may have learned. The unifying characteristic of all such processes is that they aim to demonstrate that individuals have learnt what is necessary to undertake an acceptable level of practice in their specialist area. Re-certification and re-accreditation processes have the advantage of being objective, but if they rely on formal assessment methods they can be extremely expensive if they are to be adequately robust.

Accreditation of services

Systems of health service accreditation are in widespread use throughout the world, especially in North America. Health service providers are accredited with an appropriate body in order to provide assurance for patients and for third party purchasers of healthcare that the standards within a particular provider are acceptable. It is within the capacity of any accrediting system to include standards of CPD performance within the criteria against which a particular service may be accredited.

Advantages
An assessment of compliance with predetermined standards of CPD activity is precisely the same sort of standard as others in use within the accreditation field. It can be assessed using documentary evidence.

Disadvantages
There are no specific disadvantages to using standards of CPD activity within an accreditation system. It is a feature of all such systems that they are often bureaucratic and time-consuming.

Appraisal

The best moment and technique to review the potential and actual benefits of an individual's CPD is during their appraisal meeting with a colleague. This is built into *The Good CPD Guide's* recommendations on the CPD cycle. The review of the year's activity should include a review of the CPD undertaken. This should concern:
➤ The clinician's experience of the CPD undertaken
➤ The areas where the clinician feels that he or she has benefited
➤ The areas where the clinician had hoped to gain more benefit
➤ Plans for the future.

The process of appraisal, therefore, has the capacity to judge the benefit of CPD undertaken. It is an appropriate instrument for judging the value of CPD across the full range of CPD activities.

The process of appraisal is a managed one and is generally considered valuable in all other professional areas and by doctors who are involved in such a process. The inclusion of a discussion of the value of an individual's CPD activity can easily be included with benefit to the individual and to the institution.

Appraisal might be considered to lack objectivity as a system of judging the benefits of CPD. However, in this respect, it is no different from the exercise of professional judgment in any context. A structured appraisal session can add objectivity to the process.

Assessment of learning

It is uncommon for courses to assess the learning increment enjoyed by participants, unless it is a course aimed at preparing participants for examinations. As part of their general professional development, doctors may undertake training in their specialty and in many other areas such as:

➤ Teaching skills
➤ Communication skills
➤ Team-building
➤ Management and financial skills.

Formal and informal methods may be used to assess the success of such training. There are formal instruments available to assess a doctor's interpersonal and team-related skills, such as 360° or multisource assessment or various simulations, which are often applied during or after such courses. In practice, this method may be quite widely used on an informal basis; individuals will form a judgment about whether the relevant skills have been helped by going to a relevant course. Peers will use this information to decide whether they wish to go on the same course.

Example

One health region offered a management course. The effects of the course were determined in two ways. First, an outside assessor used a semi-structured interview technique to explore the personal benefits perceived by participants. The second method used 360° appraisal. The 360° appraisal process invites colleagues to fill in a questionnaire about the individual. The colleagues are drawn from all disciplines with the intention of finding those who are senior to, junior to, and at the same level as the individual, thus gaining a view of that individual from all around. All participants arranged for a 360° appraisal process to be completed before joining the course and the results were fed back to them as part of the course. A number of participants were able to take part in a follow-up course where the 360° appraisal was repeated, thus providing a 'before and after' picture.

Assessment results of trainees

The qualities of a consultant or GP principal, as teacher and doctor, will exert some influence on the qualities and achievements of trainees. The senior must be not only a good teacher, but also demonstrate a proper role model in the practice of medicine.[51] Training in education itself is part of the range of CPD activities to be expected of a modern clinician. Likewise, changes in the clinician's practice will find their way back into the learning of the trainee. In some cases, the benefits of both may be clearly apparent in a change in the assessment performance of students and junior doctors.

Doctors in training at all levels in the UK have regular formal assessment of progress by workplace based assessments and portfolios. Doctors in training are also assessed by national postgraduate exams and this too provides evidence which may help in the evaluation of their training.

No formal methodology exists to use the wealth of data derived from the assessment of junior doctors in evaluating the clinical performance of their teachers. However, there is no reason in principle why it should not be taken advantage of and there is every reason to believe that good performance in this area would be, in part, related to enthusiastic participation in CPD by both individuals and their departments.

Advantages
Objectivity of data is a clear strength.

Disadvantages
Assessment data are not always available and might not be directly related to the areas in which the senior doctor has changed either practice or knowledge.

Audit

The memories of clinicians tend to be short and selective, and may paint a more or less favourable picture of work carried out than objective analysis can support. Audit is the objective analysis of work performed and is an essential component of CPD. This section is not concerned with the audit of CPD, but rather how clinical audit activities may be used to evaluate the effectiveness of CPD.

Audit and CPD are inextricably interlinked. The purpose of audit is to ensure the delivery of the highest possible standards of service, and the identification of these standards clearly depends in large part on the educational background of the professionals involved.

That said, it is doubtful whether serious study of the audit programme within a hospital or practice will do more than provide a picture of the general educational climate within the organisation. It seems reasonable to assert that practices, departments and hospitals which are carrying out high-quality clinical audit are also likely to be encouraging useful and appropriate CPD for their staff. It, therefore, seems reasonable to suggest that a broad-brush judgment of the audit programme within departments or whole hospitals will provide some indication of the benefits of the CPD programme that is being run. The audit programme might also, in specific circumstance, identify actual changes made as a result of CPD.

Advantages
Clinical audit activity is recorded and there are, therefore, easily accessible records on which it is possible to make a judgment of quality and enthusiasm

in the area in question. Changes in practice can also be tracked if the audit trail and the CPD coincide in content.

Disadvantages

Audits might not already cover the relevant topics undertaken in CPD. Setting up such audits might be time-consuming.

Example

An accident and emergency consultant attends a regional clinical meeting. At this meeting a colleague from another hospital presents data from a review of antibiotic use in her department. The consultant elects to audit antibiotic usage in his own department and shows that approximately one-third of all antibiotics prescribed in his department were prescribed unnecessarily. In a further one-third of patients, the choice of antibiotic was inappropriate in the opinion of a microbiologist colleague. The antibiotic of choice in this second group was invariably a narrower spectrum agent that is always cheaper. Hereafter, a policy is developed which a further audit shows has altered prescribing patterns. An inspection of this department's yearly business plan will show a record of the level of audit activity undertaken in the department. In this particular department, there is a high level of audit activity and it is of high quality. In this particular case, it would also be true to conclude that the consultant in charge of the department is committed to maintaining a high level of personal CPD.

Changes in person specification

It is now normal for new posts to be filled by a process of selection according to a predetermined person specification. The requirements of the post are determined and candidates are assessed according to the closeness with which their qualifications, skills and achievements match those of the ideal candidate described by the person specification.

Changes in person specification as result of CPD can be effected in two ways:
➤ Individuals may improve their range of skills as a result of CPD. This in turn will improve their chances of matching some potential person specifications for posts in the future
➤ As the doctors in the department improve through their CPD, the person specifications for new posts in the department will become more exciting.

This is one of the few objective measures of outcome of CPD. When an appropriate post is advertised it becomes easy to make an informed decision based upon whether individuals' educational background has equipped them with the skills specified in the person specification. As departments improve and develop, so will person specifications for posts in those departments.

Example

A physician is appointed to a hospital trust as clinical tutor with responsibility for overseeing medical education throughout the organisation. The management and educational challenges of postgraduate education prove fascinating to her, and she undertakes a wide range of CPD activities in managerial and educational areas over the next five years. She also undertakes an action research project on the introduction of service-based learning for junior medical trainees. A neighbouring trust advertises a post that is half-time in the department of medicine, and half-time as director of education for the trust. The CPD activities which she has accrued over the previous five years enable her to demonstrate that she has the skills necessary to match the person specification, and she is appointed to the new post.

Changing practice

Changes in practice should not always be expected from all CPD activity. A confirmation of current practice, which results from a genuine re-evaluation, is equally important. However, changes will often occur.

It is clear that many changes in clinical practice are brought about as a result of CPD activity. The process of cause and effect may be documented in several ways:

➤ A specific change in clinical practice can be traced retrospectively to a particular CPD episode
➤ CPD activity can be recorded and evidence for change(s) in clinical practice sought subsequently
➤ CPD and changes in practice can both be documented and collated from a single database.

This method would depend upon the generation of databases similar to those used for audit in a clinical setting or the keeping of accurate records. The method is particularly suitable for clearly defined changes in practice such as the introduction of new techniques, new drugs, new prescribing habits or new protocols which have resulted from CPD activity. It is less suitable for subtle changes in practice, and those which have come about as a result of less easily definable CPD activities such as peer discussions. Remember also, that intervening variables may hazard a positive outcome from even high-quality, well-planned CPD.

Advantages

➤ A clear relationship between certain CPD activities and changes in practice can be shown.
➤ This method can be applied to both external CPD activities and CPD activity which is internal to the hospital or practice.

Disadvantages

The effort involved in setting up databases or records which track these changes in a useful way might be substantial, so that it is unlikely that this method would be cost-effective to set up in a formal way. However, it could be undertaken informally as part of the appraisal process. The method would only identify a limited range of CPD activity.

Example

An accident and emergency consultant attends a meeting on the outpatient management of deep venous thrombosis (DVT). In his hospital, the initial investigation and treatment of patients with DVT is carried out in the accident and emergency department, but patients are traditionally admitted to hospital for further treatment. He implements a new protocol where patients are treated with once daily outpatient subcutaneous injections administered by a district nurse, prior to transfer to oral anticoagulant treatment, monitored by the out-patient haematology clinic. This outpatient treatment proves extremely popular with patients and results in a significant saving of hospital bed days. Thus, as a result of CPD, the trust experiences improved patient care and improved patient satisfaction.

Clinical effectiveness

Improved clinical effectiveness is a highly desirable key outcome of CPD, and this will have benefits for patients, individual practitioners and the health service as a whole. The basic tenet of clinical effectiveness is that patients will receive the treatment that has the greatest likelihood of producing a good outcome, and the least likelihood of producing an unfavourable or unwanted side-effect, complication or adverse effect. Clinically effective care should be a fundamental aim of all doctors and healthcare providers.

Measures of clinical effectiveness include:
➤ Mortality and morbidity studies
➤ Adverse event recording
➤ Critical incident recording
➤ Assessment of the therapeutic and interventional strategies delivered against the accepted best practice.

This method can be used in looking for improved outcome in:
➤ Individual patients
➤ Cohorts of patients with specific conditions
➤ Cohorts of patients under the care of a particular practitioner or unit
➤ Individual practitioner performance
➤ Performance of a particular cohort of doctors
➤ Range of health services available within an individual department or hospital.

Advantages

➤ This is something from the 'real world' of day-to-day clinical practice which is of central importance to all doctors.
➤ The ability to show the effectiveness of CPD in clinically relevant areas will act as positive reinforcement to individual practitioners to continue with further CPD.
➤ The same positive reinforcement will act on those responsible for funding CPD.
➤ Some of the required information may be obtainable from existing management sources.

Disadvantages

➤ Long-term, detailed collection of data will be needed if the relevant measures are to be valid and reliable.
➤ To be valid, the methodology must approach the standards of good research which may not be feasible or appropriate in many working clinical environments.

Example

In 1995, the British Cardiac Society undertook the ASPIRE study, an audit of secondary prevention in patients with ischaemic heart disease. This was a formal epidemiological study which showed that the NHS was falling well short of reasonable targets for secondary prevention activity. Because of the high quality of the data it became possible to undertake local investigation of the rate of use of secondary prevention strategies, and changes in these could be used as part of the assessment of the effectiveness of CPD in this area.

CPD credit points

Although the evidence suggests that collection of credit points for learning activity is not the most appropriate way of documenting or encouraging effective CPD, most countries with formal CPD schemes have adopted systems in which credit points are accumulated or awarded to quantify educational activities. In many schemes, such as those for most colleges in the UK, the credits are simply time-based, with one hour of real educational time equating with one credit. In other schemes, credits are weighted with more emphasis being placed on interactive education than on passive events such as lectures.

These credit-scoring systems have been generated in response to the requirement for the profession to be self-regulating and transparent. It follows that this method of recording CPD must be sufficiently robust to withstand external scrutiny. Within the profession itself, there is interest in what doctors actually do in attempting to keep up-to-date and to develop professionally.

Minimum targets have been set (50 hours per year in most colleges in the UK) with rolling programmes over five years and some form of certification of those who have satisfactorily complied with requirements at the end of that time.

Advantages

➤ Minimum targets for education are set for individual doctors.

➤ Activities can be quantified (and analysed where necessary).

➤ Participating doctors can be certificated as having their CPD 'in good standing'.

➤ A record of individual activities enables participants to plan for future CPD programmes. In the past, most doctors readily obtained their specialist educational requirements but neglected the wider aspects of professional development.

Disadvantages

➤ Activities are measured in time rather than quality.

➤ There is no evidence base that suggests how to credit-rate educational events because none is more effective than others, and each event is only predictably effective within a managed CPD system.

➤ It is difficult to equate one type of learning with another.

➤ Satisfactory completion of CPD credit requirements does not necessarily imply competence.

➤ Unnecessary bureaucracy is generated.

➤ Formal CPD departments have to be created to record data.

➤ Some doctors regard the need to record what they do as 'professionally degrading'.

➤ Some doctors may adopt the 'easy option' of undertaking all their CPD in the passive mode by attending meetings which consist of a series of lectures.

The major criticism of the credit system is that it creates an unnecessary bureaucracy and is simply 'box ticking'. Nonetheless, a formal system with 'professional obligation' creates compelling pressures on all doctors to ensure that they keep 'up-to-date' or, at least, that they attend meetings and events to gather the credit points. Those who cannot produce evidence for their CPD being of good standing may be disadvantaged medico-legally and professionally by overt or covert sanctions. This will be significant where revalidation is imposed.

Collaborative assessment

Collaborative assessment is slightly more rigorous than self-assessment (*see* below). It involves discussion and negotiation between the doctor and a colleague or senior about the goals of learning, the assessment methods and criteria, and standards to be met. This can be done in relation to any planned learning, and would fit into managed CPD and appraisal very easily. The partners can then undertake the assessment together or with the help of others.

Advantages
Collaborative assessment enhances learning and is a credible approach to deter-mining its effects.

Disadvantages
Specifying the intended outcomes of learning can sometimes limit the learner's horizons. Collaborative assessment should be limited to learning goals and events that do have a specific intended outcome.

Confidence levels

Confidence is a rather intangible quality that nevertheless underpins all that we do. It is integral to the function of senior clinicians that they are able to inter-vene decisively, not only in more complex clinical matters, but also in wider, supervisory or management areas. Without confidence, indecision, impaired effectiveness and decreased influence may result.

Clinicians who are up-to-date with their subject, and know they are, will be confident in less familiar situations; being aware of personal limitations in knowledge or skill, and they will be able to act accordingly in the interests of the patient. Confidence similarly enhances the collaboration with patients in selecting the most appropriate treatment or management.

Confidence is generally perceived to be a positive attribute. However, over-confidence, particularly when associated with a lack of insight, can be dangerous. The recognition of the limits of an individual's experience and knowledge is a determining characteristic of high-quality professional behaviour. A good pro-fessional will be well aware that it is possible to acquire limited knowledge and skill through CPD which may be inadequate for the task in hand.

No validated tests exist to assess clinical confidence. One must rely on sub-jective measures or develop new ones. Confidence must be something felt by the individual, and may be increased by the belief that the knowledge gained is valuable. Exploration of these areas is an appropriate part of any appraisal or reporting back process.

Confidence in the knowledge or skills gained from CPD can be reinforced by teaching. Routine presentations after CPD activity can therefore help to bolster the confidence of an individual professional who has been away at a meeting or a course, while the quality of that professional's presentation may give some indication of the confidence-enhancing qualities of the CPD which they have undertaken while reinforcing its educative effect.

Corporate image

CPD enhances the skills and knowledge of consultants, general practitioners and others in career posts, but it may do so in an intangible way. This makes sub-stantial expenditure hard to justify. However, the image of the trust or primary care group as a provider of high-quality care and a site of learning is important.

In this instance, CPD is an important part of the public relations effort of the organisation.

Effects on the public image of the organisation can be in terms of the educational profile of all doctors in the organisation and the consequent quality of the service they provide.

Although the organisation will be concerned to promote its external image, its image to those who work within it is just as important. All employees derive satisfaction from knowing that the work their organisation is engaged in is of very high quality and is recognised as such by outside observers. In practices, hospitals and trusts where there is a justified self-image of high quality, the prophecy seems to become self-fulfilling.

An effective communications department within a hospital trust or primary care group will keep up-to-date with the activities of its staff who promote its image as a learned and high-quality institution.

Advantages and disadvantages

Any judgment of image, be it the external image or that perceived from the inside, is necessarily subjective. However, such judgments can be elicited formally through surveys and questionnaires.

Example

A Trust Chief Executive sees that there is little to attract high-quality staff to his hospital. The surroundings are those of a faded industrial landscape. There is strong academic competition from the local teaching hospital. Nevertheless, he recognises and encourages the enthusiasm and academic potential of the paediatric department and of two consultants in the department of anaesthesia. Over five years, four of his consultants become well-known nationally and he sees the benefits in terms of improved recruitment to these two hard-pressed units. Stronger links with the local university are set up and two or three joint appointments are made which should serve to strengthen other departments.

Decreasing professional isolation

Doctors in the career grades may easily suffer from isolation, either as a result of geography or because they are in a small specialty or single-handed practice and are therefore working alone much of the time. The educational culture of geographically isolated hospitals and of departments and practices where there are single-handed doctors is therefore especially important.

However, for those who are both geographically isolated and in a small specialty, there are particular problems and there seems no avoiding the need to travel to maintain a professional identity by contact with colleagues at meetings and on learning visits to bigger departments, although distance learning methods and communication technologies can also be used to interact with colleagues.

The risks of professional isolation are clear to those who are at risk. The evaluation of the benefits of CPD will depend upon the extent to which isolated practitioners and their management teams feel that the problem is being avoided. An evaluation of the degree of professional isolation can be undertaken by reporting to colleagues, and by identifying the professional contacts that have been established and maintained.

The avoidance of professional isolation is of great importance to both the doctors and the patients whom they serve. Attention to this outcome is therefore important. The fact that the judgments reached will often be subjective does not diminish the importance of the outcome.

'Don't know' factor

One important characteristic of confident clinicians, is the ability to recognise the limits of their knowledge and to say, 'I don't know'. Curiously, those who are most experienced and knowledgeable seem most able to say, 'I don't know', while those whose clinical skills are less securely founded are perhaps more inclined to prevaricate. Some would regard this as the touchstone of clinical wisdom.

From an institutional perspective, a judgment that senior clinicians are prepared to say, 'I don't know', is a good indicator of the presence of a climate of openness within the institution. It would be quite inappropriate to use some objective test of the borders of ignorance as a measure of clinical wisdom. Nevertheless the ability to say, 'I don't know' when it is appropriate to do so, is an important element in the judgments of professional skill made by doctors about their colleagues. It is probably most important when junior colleagues are judging the skills of their seniors. It follows that a judgment of this ability could be used to assess the overall state of clinicians' clinical confidence, which in turn provides an indication of the success of their CPD to date and also their needs for the future.

A perceived lack of an ability to say, 'I don't know' indicates the need to work on an individual's clinical confidence, and CPD planning should be directed to this end.

Educational culture

The management teams of all sorts of different organisations are increasingly realising that, to be successful, they must have a workforce who continue to learn and develop during their professional lives. This is no less the case in hospitals and other organisations which provide healthcare. A major purpose of CPD is to promote the overall climate of education and enhance patient care within an organisation. However, one of the major goals for organisations over the next few years will be to make sure that the promotion and support of education extends to all other workers within the organisation. Many trusts and practices are making great efforts to promote the educational activities of nurses and other professional staff; however, the challenge lies just as much in the promotion of training and development among the non-professional workers.

The rationale for this approach lies in the fact that appropriate, enthusiastic involvement in educational activity by clinicians is an important catalyst to promote commitment to training everywhere else in the organisation. In this instance, subjective judgment is less than satisfactory. For example, as a medical director catches sight of the clinical tutor snatching a brief conversation with a junior between clinics, it is all too easy for him to convince himself that there is a strong educational climate within the hospital. To demonstrate the presence of such a climate, it is necessary to demonstrate that the organisational infrastructure exists to support widespread educational activity.

In hospitals with a strong educational culture, individuals have specific responsibilities to promote training and personal development for all staff. Such individuals should have time within their contract to work on providing the support that is needed to promote training and development. There should also be explicit written policies which deal with such activities as study leave for junior doctors and CPD for career-grade staff.

This is an approach which needs to be part of the overall management view of education and training. There should be trust-wide policies for CPD. The same applies to primary care groups.

Advantages and disadvantages
CPD activity is only one of the elements of medical life which leads to a vigorous educational culture. It is perhaps more pertinent to say that where such a culture is not demonstrable, there may also be problems with the promotion and uptake of effective CPD.

Educational records and log-books

As part of the implementation of formal CPD schemes, paper or electronic log-books or diaries are often used in which consultants and those in the other career grades can record their educational activities, as part of their portfolio. These records are often designed to allow analysis of doctors' CPD into various categories and to enable the supervising organisation to establish whether the basic (time-based) educational targets are being achieved.

While filling in log-books is regarded by most doctors as a bureaucratic chore, professional organisations have a self-regulatory function to ensure that they have records of what doctors actually do. Unfortunately, the entries are difficult to validate and their owners do not necessarily fill them in on a day-to-day basis. They also only record attendance at events rather than their quality or outcome.

Nevertheless, they enable doctors to assess what they are doing with their valuable study time and to define patterns of work. They may reveal, for example, undue emphasis on specialist clinical work and insufficient attention to wider professional responsibilities such as management, finance, audit and inter-professional working.

Log-books do serve as a record of CPD activity, but they are appropriate only to those areas of formal CPD which are recognised as entities.

Advantages
➤ The log-books/diaries are small, simple to complete and comprehensive for those events they cover.
➤ They contain a time-based record of education.
➤ They indicate the proportion of internal (home-based) CPD to external CPD (for which study leave is required).
➤ Specific categories of educational activity are recorded.
➤ They enable the doctor to review the allocation of this study time.
➤ They are chronologically-based.
➤ They can be audited if necessary.

Disadvantages
➤ They are bureaucratic.
➤ They are seen as a chore to complete.
➤ Some events are forgotten.
➤ The credit scoring is time-based rather than quality controlled.
➤ Their completion depends on the honesty of the owner.
➤ Many educational 'events' such as professional conversations, reflective learning and learning from mistakes are not included.
➤ Satisfactory 'time-based' education does not guarantee competence.

Effects on the team

Patient care is now largely team-based. If CPD is to have useful benefits for patient care it will also have useful benefits for the team. External peer review looks at this aspect. Other methods might also be used to demonstrate the benefits of CPD to the team. The factors these methods might address include:
➤ A better team as a result of a better informed and skilled team leader
➤ A greater pool of knowledge which is then shared
➤ Consultants who make efforts to pursue their own education act as role models
➤ Teams in which continuing education is valued, act as role models for other teams
➤ Teams with a leader who is committed to CPD will attract high-quality team members.

The increasing importance of teams is highlighted by the fact that national awards now exist for teams in various disciplines. Teams provide an excellent setting for the use of formal 360° appraisal methods, and instruments could be developed to look at the potential benefits listed above. Data could be gathered by means of questionnaires, interview studies or rating scales. It would then be possible to compare the performance of teams judged to have a high level of CPD activity among its leaders with other teams judged to have a lower level of activity.

Advantages

It would be desirable for any system of managed CPD to take note of the impact that CPD has on the function of teams, especially where multiprofessional working is fundamental to patient care.

Disadvantages

This approach would lend itself to the development of formal instruments to study the effects of CPD on teams. These would have to be developed and administered.

Enhancing practice

New information and new techniques are appearing constantly, producing a change in the way clinical practice is carried out. The relentless onward march of information and technology can appear in one of two ways to a career-grade doctor. It can be seen in a positive light as a way of enhancing clinical practice. For such doctors, enhancing clinical practice also enhances their own satisfaction and enthusiasm. Another doctor in another place may see the advances as a threat and a further contribution to the feeling that he or she is dropping behind. A major purpose of ensuring that all career-grade staff have a programme of CPD is to make sure that as many people as possible take the optimistic and enthusiastic view of advances in information and technology.

Enhancing practice will also have the positive effects of reinforcing the learning by using it and of disseminating that learning to colleagues through planning and implementation of an innovation.

Individual doctors should reflect on technological and other developments and their attitudes towards them. In many cases, they will regard it as essential to take on a new development to provide the best possible service for the patients for whom they are responsible. In such circumstances, it is vital to ensure that the relevant education and understanding are acquired (along with any new equipment that may be involved).

Such reflection by the individual may also form part of appraisal. Improving the quality of patient care is not only a valuable end in itself but is also an enriching experience for all doctors. Knowledge and technology are advancing in all areas of medicine, with the opportunity to make continuous improvements. On the other side of the coin, it is also true to say that all doctors may be vulnerable to feelings of inadequacy if they fear that knowledge and technology are advancing beyond the horizon of their understanding.

The enthusiasm with which older doctors embrace changes in clinical practice acts as a measure of their morale and job satisfaction. It is therefore an important area of enquiry. It remains an area of professional judgment but is no less valuable for that.

Example

Laparoscopic surgery is an excellent example of a change in technology that produced differing reactions among practitioners. Some embraced it enthusiastically, but did not undertake additional training. Others hung back and found the new developments threatening, and some embraced the new technology with the necessary training to go with it. Following up such innovations with discussion of how it enhances or even detracts from practice, could be very helpful for the whole team.

Learning diaries

A learning diary is a written or computerised record of learning which serves to demonstrate how, when and what learning has occurred, as well as reinforcing that learning by promoting further thought about it and how it might affect practice. A learning diary has the strength of being able to contain details of informal and opportunistic learning, such as discussion with colleagues. Diaries can be written freehand or structured under various headings such as:

➤ Date
➤ What was learned?
➤ How it was learned?
➤ Likely effect on practice/value of the learning.

Some specialties have designed and evaluated diaries that are more complex.

Learning portfolios

A learning portfolio is a comprehensive record of learning events, along with evidence of outcomes. This is likely to be a component of revalidation procedures, in some form. It is an extension of the learning diary and contains not only the diary record, but also such documents as:

➤ Log-books
➤ Research undertaken
➤ Research proposals
➤ Clinical data
➤ Jottings (ideas, thoughts, insights, challenges)
➤ A reflective commentary in which the individual identifies what has been learned.

The portfolio provides a way of assessing professional development by gathering together documents, new protocols, audit data, research reports and so on, in a way that is open to scrutiny. Headings in the portfolio can include:

➤ Structured/organised training
➤ Learning on the job
➤ Learning off the job
➤ Professional activities
➤ Informal learning.

The portfolio is thus a way of encouraging, structuring, recording and reflecting on the learning that arises from practice and formal events.

Advantages
A learning portfolio has the advantage of comprehensiveness. It is capable of containing all the data and records that are relevant to formal continuing learning. It can also show how that learning is applied to practice and is an open and accessible record.

Disadvantages
The portfolio can be time-consuming to construct and organise. It will also be time-consuming to assess or review. Little is known about the reliability of learning portfolios, although face-validity is high.

New services
Hospitals or practices setting up a new service are involved in a relatively high order of change. A business case needs to be made for a new service upon which funding can be based. The existence of the new service needs to be made known both within and outside the hospital. Many new services are set up as a direct result of the gains in knowledge and understanding produced by CPD.

A hospital trust might choose to look at any new service that has been set up within the previous year in making an annual assessment of the overall benefits of its CPD programme. Those involved in making the assessment would then be able to make a judgment of the part the CPD programme had played in leading to the establishment of such new services as they can identify.

Advantages
New services are easy to identify because considerable management effort is involved in setting them up.

Disadvantages
It is difficult to disentangle the many forces for change which may lead to a new service being set up. CPD activity will be only one of these forces.

Example
The creation of a rapid access service for patients with acute low back pain is an example. This service was developed in accordance with currently accepted guidelines on the management of acute low back pain. The emphasis was on triage, rapid mobilisation and rehabilitation, the use of non-medical healthcare

personnel (for example, physiotherapists) and the total avoidance of referral of patients to rheumatology or orthopaedic specialists unless a well-defined indication was identified. The pressure for change leading to the development of the service resulted from the continuing professional education of physiotherapists and the CPD activities of pain specialists, rheumatologists, orthopaedic surgeons and local general practitioners.

Obsolete and inappropriate practice

Effective CPD should lead to the adoption of clinical practices for which there exists positive evidence of clinical effectiveness, and the abandonment of clinical practices which are inappropriate. Such practices may have been shown to lack clinical effectiveness, or there may be an unacceptably high incidence of adverse events. This benefit can be demonstrated by comparing the present rate of an obsolete or inappropriate clinical practice with a known previous rate. Effective CPD should also lead to the decrease of broader organisational practices in medical care where there is poor cost-effectiveness, diminished efficiency or inappropriateness. Information can be gleaned from many sources and these include:

➤ Audit of practitioner/departmental activity
➤ Operating theatre records
➤ Prescribing records generated by pharmacy
➤ Hospital or practice purchasing records for drugs or equipment
➤ Records of investigations ordered.

This method could be applied widely throughout clinical practice, including individual patient care, patterns of care and aspects of organisation. Areas of potential interest include:

➤ Referral patterns: Are general practitioners (and hospital doctors) making appropriate referrals?
➤ Organisation: Are practices or hospital clinics clinging to obsolete or outmoded organisational arrangements? This includes things such as the ability to retrieve and access patient records, appropriate use of information technology and adequacy of communication and follow-up arrangements.
➤ Investigations: Are doctors ordering unnecessary, inappropriate or obsolete investigations?
➤ Treatment: Are doctors prescribing or performing treatments which are known to be ineffective or associated with an unacceptably high incidence of adverse events?

Advantages
➤ A reduction of obsolete or inappropriate practice is clear evidence of improving clinical effectiveness. The method relies on the demonstration of change in practice and is therefore good evidence of educational effect. There is also:

 – positive risk management implications for the practitioner and the
    practice or hospital
 – positive feedback to managers, clinical directors and purchasers.

Disadvantages

Decreased use of an obsolete practice may have occurred because of factors
other than CPD, such as pressure by purchasers, lack of funds, alteration in the
availability of a particular drug or the availability of particular equipment. There
may be disagreement as to whether the clinical practice is really obsolete or
inappropriate, especially if powerful voices are raised in defence of the practice.

Peer review of the medical team

Peer review visits may focus on the work of the medical team as a whole, rather
than on the work of an individual clinician. However, such occasions can also
be used to determine the effects of CPD undertaken. The visiting peer reviewers
can look especially at those areas in which CPD has been undertaken and to the
dissemination of CPD from individual clinicians to the whole medical team, as
an indication of effectiveness.

Personal invigoration

There is often much truth in platitudes: variety really is the spice of life!
Motivation is essential if CPD is to have positive benefits on practice and on
personal wellbeing. One of the most common, but least tangible benefits of
CPD is a sense of renewed enthusiasm. This is seen even if the CPD activity is
only peripherally relevant to day-to-day concerns. By being able to take time out
from clinical duties and to experience an educational environment that stretches
the mind, a doctor can return stimulated and able to place day-to-day concerns
in context. When doctors take part in CPD this is an indication that they value
themselves; this too, can have an invigorating effect.

  Personal invigoration is, of course, subjective. This does not mean that a
scale could not be developed and validated to measure it.

Protection from successful litigation

Accumulated case law in England and Wales has tended to support the notion
that practice is not negligent if it is consistent with the practice followed by a
'substantial' body of 'reputable' practitioners. Thus, a practitioner accused of
negligence can mount a vigorous defence if one or more experts are prepared to
attest that the procedures which were followed are widely accepted. The problem with this is that established patterns of practice are hard to define and courts
may be left with the choice of which expert testimony they prefer. While it may
be the case that most doctors can identify practice which is obviously eccentric
or inappropriate, it may be more difficult in complex cases where deviation
from some proposed standard of care is more subtle. The question is whether a

doctor who could show that his record of CPD was up-to-date would add more strength to his argument that the episode of care which led to the allegation of negligence was, in fact, reasonable.

Complementing this, the doctor who is fully involved in CPD may well find that the threat and actuality of litigation subside. Few doctors would wish to be a successful defendant in order to demonstrate the benefits of CPD. However, doctors might reflect on rates of actual and likely litigation and means of protecting themselves from this.

Recruitment of medical staff

The single most powerful argument for an active CPD programme that is encouraged and managed by a supportive organisation is the effect on the recruitment and the retention of staff. High-quality, career-grade staff are attracted to organisations which have a well-developed, educational culture. There is also a virtuous circle operating on the interdependent effects of consultant recruitment and the attraction of training-grade staff to the hospital. This has been termed the 'cascade of benefits':

- A better educational environment attracts
- High-quality doctors who attract
- Higher calibre doctors in training, who (with their seniors) produce
- Higher quality clinical care and research, which attracts
- More high-quality doctors, which produces
- A higher quality educational environment

Figure 6: The cascade of benefits

There are many different ways of writing down such cascades or virtuous circles, but the principle remains the same: high-quality medical staff are attracted to work in organisations which are committed to education.

This is a method which can be employed every time a post is advertised or training is applied for. If the standards of the applicants are increasing it suggests that the educational reputation of the hospital and the relevant department is rising.

Advantages
➤ Hospitals are appointing doctors all the time, so it is always possible to make a judgment about the relative attractiveness of a given hospital.

➤ Variation between hospitals and the perceived educational benefits which they offer is probably one of the most important factors influencing junior staff in applying for training rotations.

Disadvantages
➤ The timescale of the effect of the educational environment is long. Departmental reputations are built in quinquennia, not mere years. Sustained efforts by consultants and departments may be needed before there is a discernible effect on recruitment.

Reduction in burnout and early retirement
In a hard-pressed, service-orientated post, the insidious signs of loss of interest and enthusiasm, dread of going to work, increased irritability and superficial assessment of problems are all harbingers of burnout. The affected doctor may have a sense of being both undervalued and overwhelmed. Sometimes clinical depression may supervene. Such doctors may retire early or simply leave their post.

While the loss of medical workforce to the NHS through early retirement is a cause of concern, those doctors who fail to take any action and simply struggle on may cause even greater problems to themselves, their patients and employers. The problems of both early retirement and burnout of senior clinical staff are a major problem for the NHS and anything which will reduce the level of these problems must be encouraged.

Medicine is a career where there is abundant fascination but also abundant challenge. When these two forces become out of equilibrium and challenge becomes a threat while enthusiasm and fascination decline, then burnout becomes a very real danger.

The benefit of CPD is simple. In this most fascinating of disciplines, continuing education breeds continuing enthusiasm for the subject. The level of early retirements will provide an indication of the overall enthusiasm of the workforce. Burnout may be more difficult to identify, but questionnaires exist, of which one of the best known is the Maslach Burnout Inventory.*

To identify a doctor who is already suffering from burnout is to act too late. The process of appraisal which is integral to managed CPD, should be used to identify problems early. Individual doctors might be asked to reflect on how they feel each evening before work. Do they dread the next day (and perhaps drink to numb the pain)? Or are they excited by the challenge?

Advantages
Anything which encourages doctors themselves and those who manage them to concentrate on maintaining their health and enthusiasm is to be encouraged.

---

*www.mindtools.com/stress/Brn/BurnoutSelfTest.htm

Disadvantages

While the level of early retirement and burnout are likely to be rather an accurate yardstick for the level of clinical enthusiasm within an organisation, this method of assessing the benefits of CPD is likely to remain subjective, since the use of scale-based measures of burnout would be likely to be perceived as impersonal and intimidating as well as possibly stigmatising.

Example

Happily, there are now many examples of management teams which take these problems very seriously. Of those that do, it may be that only a minority realise the contribution that well-managed CPD can make to minimising this problem.

Referrals to the doctor

Consultants who keep up-to-date with their field through CPD may have an increased referral rate to them. This variable can be investigated by:
- ➤ Looking at referral patterns for individual consultants and comparing it with their CPD activity
- ➤ Surveys. A questionnaire study of GPs, for example, may reveal that some consultants are regarded as more up-to-date in their field than others.

Advantages and disadvantages

The factors governing a GP's decision to refer to a particular hospital and to a particular consultant are complex. The effect that consultant CPD may have on this decision is likely to be confounded by other variables. There is also a problem with the halo effect. Consultants who keep up-to-date with their CPD are likely to have other positive traits which are not directly related to CPD. Finally, in the modern era there are a relatively low number of consultants who do not keep up with their CPD; so an increased referral rate as a result of enthusiastic participation in CPD can only be relative and there will be few consultants perceived to be sub-optimal in this respect. However, a consideration of the CPD activity of those few consultants who do have low referral rates may suggest a perception that such consultants do not keep up-to-date may be part of the problem.

Remunerative benefit

One of the ways in which consultants and other career-grade staff may benefit from CPD is by increasing their earnings. There are a number of ways in which this might happen:
- ➤ Faster progression up the salary scale. The acquisition of a higher degree or valuable skill might lead to a consultant (or other career-grade doctor) moving up more than one annual increment on the salary scale
- ➤ Writing. People who become involved in the academic side of their discipline may get involved in writing articles for the professional and lay press which in turn may produce a small income through fees and speaking invitations

➤ Paid lectureships, travelling fellowships etc. People who become involved in the academic side of their discipline may then start to earn the honoraria which accompany lecturing and other such activities. It must be said that the amounts involved are small, but this is the sort of activity which may lead on to the award of discretionary points and merit awards

➤ The earlier acquisition of discretionary points and merit awards. Merit awards and discretionary points are now awarded in a way that is much more transparent than hitherto. The criteria for selection are published and criteria such as audit and research clearly depend upon CPD activity, especially where individuals do not have a formal academic commitment within their contract. Activity in the areas of service development, teaching and the wider contribution to the health service may also be strongly rooted in an individual's CPD activity

➤ Remuneration in private practice. CPD may benefit a consultant's private practice as much as his or her NHS practice

➤ Medico-legal work. CPD activity may support a consultant's medico-legal activities.

The earnings and advances are clear and can be measured. It may be more difficult to reach a complete judgment about the contribution that CPD has made. Nonetheless, a professional judgment can be made quite effectively. This method is clearly helpful for individuals to make judgments about their own CPD. For NHS employers, this method may be useful since the number of higher award holders may be thought to reflect the prestige of the institution.

It might be thought that the external earnings of individuals would be of little interest to an NHS institution, but a well-managed trust or primary care group will always have the interests of its doctors (including their earning capacity) at heart – provided there is no conflict with the prime task of providing patient care.

Reporting back to colleagues

It should be regarded as a professional responsibility to colleagues and employer, after attending a CPD function, to report back to the appropriate professional group. Such reporting consolidates the educational gains for the individual clinician and helps to disseminate new knowledge and understanding within the organisation.

Although bringing new learning back to colleagues could take the form of a written report of CPD, a presentation at a regular departmental meeting or even a separate meeting convened solely for the purpose is likely to be much more effective. It has the advantage of interaction with, and feedback from, other members of the department which makes it much more likely that everyone benefits from the process.

In one form or another, the method is suitable for most CPD activities, but is particularly valuable for external meetings such as national and international conferences and symposia. CPD activities involving skills training may not be so well suited to feedback in a formal setting, although it may still be appropriate to discuss the possible impact of newly acquired skills and techniques during a departmental meeting.

Example

An example might be that a consultant surgeon attends the annual conference of the National Association of Surgeons. At this conference, which lasts three days, 120 short papers across a wide range of subspecialties within the generality of surgery are presented. A study leave form, submitted to the clinical director of surgery and then the clinical tutor, notes that the conference attracts 15 CPD credits and that the surgeon has undertaken to present a synopsis to the monthly surgical CPD meeting on a specified date. At this meeting attended by general as well as specialist surgeons, the programme is circulated in the form of a hand-out and highlights presented. Interactive discussion follows.

Advantages

➤ Maximises the value of hard-pressed study leave budgets.
➤ Renders the process and content of CPD transparent.
➤ By imposing the discipline of attendance, concentration, reflection, recall, analysis and presentation it enhances the learning experience for the individual.
➤ New knowledge is disseminated more efficiently within the institution and by placing it in context for that institution, department or clinical team, the reporter may well be able to add local knowledge and understanding to new information.
➤ Provides the opportunity for interdisciplinary CPD within the hospital or Directorate.
➤ Interactive rather than written reporting enhances understanding and transmission.
➤ Provides material by which the individual can demonstrate that he or she is undertaking CPD.
➤ Provides a further opportunity for debate.
➤ It can be argued that a responsibility to disseminate new knowledge and understanding within an institution goes hand in hand with a right to CPD.

Disadvantages

There are few disadvantages of the method although it could be argued that a significant, extra burden of work is placed on the doctor undergoing CPD.

Reputation as a trainer

The onward dissemination of knowledge and understanding is an essential part of the backdrop to CPD. For many doctors, CPD is as important to them in fulfilling their role as a trainer as it is in fulfilling their role as a clinician. It is particularly relevant to the transmission of new knowledge from the cutting edge of medicine.

CPD concerns the individual. However, CPD has its greatest value when new knowledge can be passed on to others for their benefit and for the benefit of the clinical team, the department and the hospital at large. All CPD can and should relate to trainees. CPD is important for rapid dissemination of knowledge to trainees. The reputation of consultants and of departments for teaching and training may rest in large part upon their CPD activities and their capacity to turn that experience into valuable education for others. The converse also applies; consultants may be unpopular as trainers and this may in part be due to deficiencies in their own continuing education and development.

There can be few forms of CPD where the potential benefits do not extend to an improvement in teaching and training.

Advantages

Experience suggests that the informal evaluation of the training ability of both individuals and departments is widely used as a surrogate for overall professional quality. Using trainees' evaluations of teaching could be a powerful demonstration of the effect of CPD in the department. In the UK, the GMC conducts a trainee survey on an annual basis.

Disadvantages

Trainees are not always willing to give their true opinion of their teachers and gathering information about educational reputation informally must often be an opportunistic process.

Example

There are gaps in the local specialist training scheme for rheumatology. More optional posts exist than funded trainees to fill them. A trainee is in discussion with his programme director and she is offered a choice between a post at Hospital A and a post at Hospital B. She knows both the consultants at Hospital A because she has seen them both present data at national meetings. They both have the reputation as good teachers who retain their interest and enthusiasm for their subject. In the course of conversation with peers at the last national meeting she had asked to have the consultants from Hospital B pointed out to her. As a result, she learned that the consultants rarely, if ever, went to meetings. Unsurprisingly, she opts to undertake her next year of training in Hospital A.

Research

Effective CPD should produce enhanced knowledge, enhanced skills and, very importantly, enhanced understanding and confidence. Greater knowledge and understanding should allow the doctor greater facility in identifying pertinent research questions in the doctor's domain of clinical practice.

The generation of publications or presentations at meetings not only provides concrete evidence of CPD activity but also enhances the reputation of the individual, the department and the whole institution.

The benefit of CPD to new research could be demonstrated at an individual, departmental or institutional level by assessing both the quantity and quality of the research produced. Details of publications and presentations of research projects should be recorded, although care must be taken to avoid giving too much weight to numbers of publications when analysing research activity: quality and clinical relevance must be considered as well. Due notice should be taken of the doctor who is stimulated to undertake some relatively low-key piece of research when there is no particular published record of involvement in research by that individual or institution. Such research may not reach national or international publication, but the fact that any research is occurring in a particular place may in itself have important consequences for CPD among staff not immediately involved in the project.

Those who undertake research might be asked to identify the factors which influenced each of their research projects. This could be done at the time ethical approval is sought. When an individual (or research team) applies for ethical approval for a particular research project, the application might include a statement about the influence of CPD. For example, was this idea generated as a result of attendance at meetings, or by discussion with colleagues or by reading other papers? The questions should refer to CPD influences on:

➤ The genesis of the research question
➤ The research methods
➤ The analysis of the data
➤ The literature review and generation of the discussion.

An analysis of new research will not be an appropriate measure for every doctor or in every institution. It is probably of greatest value in assessing the overall academic climate in those hospitals not traditionally associated with a large research output.

Advantages

There is a virtuous circularity in the use of the evaluation of research activity in order to evaluate CPD activity. The underlying rationale is that CPD leads to increased understanding, and that increased understanding leads to the interest and enthusiasm to carry out research and the ability to generate the ideas upon which the research may be based. Therefore, it should be possible to evaluate the CPD activities of an individual or department by counting the quantity of research produced and paying due heed to its quality.

The process of involvement in research of itself has great educational benefit to individuals because:

➤ The doctor will have to read, critically appraise and summarise existing knowledge gleaned from the medical literature in order to design and write up the project

➤ Participation in research is usually collaborative and this will allow discussion, comparison and critical analysis of such differences in clinical practice as exists amongst the various participants

➤ Research activity is often contagious or at least it heightens awareness of problems, raises questions and stimulates discussion with colleagues and other staff who are not immediately involved in the project.

Disadvantages

➤ It may be difficult to establish just how influential CPD has been in the genesis or completion of a particular research project. Much research is undertaken at the request of third parties rather than as a result of an individual's CPD activity.

➤ If research was accorded too much prominence as a good measure of CPD, it may add undesirable emphasis to the idea that a long list of publications is a reliable indication of clinical abilities. In fact, clinical abilities must be judged in a much broader context.

➤ The ability, funding and facilities to perform research are not readily available to every doctor or in every institution.

Risk management

All UK hospital trusts are now obliged to develop a clinical risk management strategy. This has four major components:

➤ Prevention – research, evidence-based practice, guidelines and protocols

➤ Reporting systems – audit, identification of risk or poor practice, remedial action, learning from mistakes

➤ Risk profile analysis and assessment – common themes and major problems, assessment methodology

➤ Claims management.

Because of its intimate involvement in the first three components, CPD can be the progenitor or the product of clinical risk management. For example, clinicians may learn of more effective treatments or clinical pathways at a meeting; conversely, the demonstration of poor practice may identify an educational need.

Clinical risk management has close links to the development of good and effective clinical practice, and is part of clinical governance. The Government's increasing emphasis on the personal responsibility of trust chief executives for this area should help to move CPD significantly up the agenda of trusts.

The benefits of CPD may be explored by:

➤ Monitoring the number of complaints
➤ Critical incident surveys
➤ Surveys of patient satisfaction.

Advantages
This method uses data that are already collected by trusts or practices. There is a rising tide of complaint and medical negligence litigation, and data should probably be considered in terms of a reduction in the rate of increase rather than reductions in the absolute number of complaints and episodes of litigation.

Disadvantages
It is well known that patient complaints arise more often from difficulties in communication across a range of staff. Complaints about isolated lapses of competence by medical staff are, in fact, rather rare. Considering CPD along with the results of critical incident data may be more informative.

Example
A trust asks the hospital solicitor to present a series of meetings at the multi-disciplinary grand round. The solicitor is an effective presenter. Staff of a variety of different disciplines from many different departments attend. The Chief Executive and the Medical Director feel that there is an increased awareness in two important areas: issues of consent and the importance of maintaining complete records. It will take a year or two to see if this intervention is effective in stemming the rising tide of litigation being experienced by this hospital and those around it.

Self-assessment

Independent practitioners in any profession must develop the skills of self-assessment. Although we must be aware that this is limited in its validity and reliability.[31] On a daily basis, there are few other ways of knowing that personal performance is adequate. Self-assessment skills range from the light end of the scale represented by the habits of the 'reflective practitioner' who incorporates into his practice an on-going and constant review of that practice and its out-comes. The term 'reflective practitioner' describes most professionals. However, self-assessment can be extended to a more formal process which is capable of being presented either at appraisal or to colleagues in the department.

Self-assessment involves the following steps which can be implemented in relation to any CPD event:

➤ Setting personal goals for the CPD
➤ Monitoring one's work against personally set criteria deriving from those goals
➤ Judging the final outcome.

This may well be the most elegant and necessary form of assessment for a professional. But its limitations must be recognised.

Advantages
➤ Self-assessment causes the individual to think seriously and realistically about the education being planned and what benefit is likely to be gained from it.
➤ Setting goals for education often encourages the learner to seek the experiences that will fulfil those goals, thus enhancing and focusing the learning.
➤ It is a rational process which matches very well with the professional approach to practice. It will reinforce positive attitudes towards learning and its integration with practice.
➤ Self-assessment, if conducted as described, can be reported to colleagues or employers.

Disadvantages
There are disadvantages to self-assessment.
➤ It might seem subjective to the psychometrically minded, but it is amenable to external checking.
➤ The doctor must be organised to implement self-assessment – but it is not very time-consuming.
➤ It does lack reliability and validity if it is seen as a true assessment rather than an analytical reflection on practice.

Time-efficient working
CPD is seen as a means of maintaining and increasing the quality of professional care. The efficiency of care is an element of quality and improvement in the use of doctors' and other health workers' time that may come about as a result of CPD activity or similar professional development activities by managers, nurses and other groups. There may also be clear improvements in efficiency of the service as a result of better matching of tasks to the skills of those providing them.

Such changes in working practices are also a reinforcement of the learning undertaken.

Example
In the 1970s and early 1980s many diabetologists attended courses in patient education. The few diabetic specialist nurses who were in post at the time also attended the same courses. This CPD activity was the major motivational force behind the drive to appoint such nurses in hospitals. This produced some saving in consultant time and, more importantly, produced a good match between the skills of the nurses and the task of patient education.

Video assessment

This method can be used for showing that change has occurred as a result of CPD, if recordings are available before and after the CPD in question. If not, video tapes can be used to demonstrate to colleagues and to discuss with them whatever has been learned through CPD.

Written reports

A major focus of CPD is the development or education of the individual. But the implications of CPD extend beyond that to the team, department and institution. Some CPD events may have considerable financial implications for the employers. Even where an employer is not paying for a particular CPD activity, there is still an opportunity cost to be borne. It is therefore quite reasonable that employers should be able to know what they have been paying for. On these grounds alone, it is reasonable for some form of formal reporting of CPD. In practice, of course, there is much to be gained by using departmental meetings and other meetings to report back on CPD, thus allowing the benefits of new knowledge and understanding to be disseminated through the organisation (*see* 'Reporting Back to Colleagues', above).

An appropriate written reporting system could be based upon:

➤ A statement of the overall content and structure of the meeting, perhaps including a copy of the programme
➤ A summary of the main points that were learned
➤ Applicability of what was learned to the doctor and the department
➤ An overall evaluation of the meeting.

The report should be circulated to colleagues, the CPD appraiser, college tutor and other interested individuals, perhaps for later discussion at an agreed time. This form of reporting back might be most appropriate for external CPD where participants have attended national or international meetings or even skills training courses.

Advantages

➤ Written reports of meetings provide a database for the future. Those planning CPD for a department may be able to use these records to decide the relative value of various meetings and courses.
➤ Written reports provide documentation to demonstrate the effective management of CPD.

Disadvantages

It is unlikely that clinicians will warm to the task of writing these reports since they are likely to be seen as a bureaucratic exercise.

Appendix 1: Overview of the literature*

CONTENTS

*Based on *The Effectiveness of Continuing Professional Development*. J Grant and F Stanton. Association for the Study of Medical Education, 2000. ISBN 0-9044-73260.

1 INTRODUCTION

The challenge of providing an evidential basis about the effectiveness of continuing professional development is considerable. As with research into education in general, the evidence is often weak and inconclusive. Nonetheless, there are some highly significant messages which indicate positive ways ahead. These messages are substantial enough to pool together and offer a foundation for subsequent strategy.

> The main message to emerge is that the key to life-long, effective learning is not to be found in advice about how to learn but rather in how to manage the learning process.

Continuing professional development (CPD) is concerned with the acquisition, enhancement and maintenance of knowledge, skills and attitudes by professional practitioners, and its broad aims are to enhance professionals' performance and optimise the outcomes of their practice. For the European Union of Medical Specialists, continuing professional development is:

> 'The educative means of updating, developing and enhancing how doctors apply the knowledge, skills and attitudes required in their working lives. The UEMS therefore believe that CPD is essential for ensuring high standards of medical practice.'

CPD is a fundamental part of professional life and a means of sustaining the workforce (Curran *et al.*, 2010). The purpose of this paper is to review the recent literature in this area to discover the relative effectiveness of different CPD activities, in terms of the achievement of the aims of CPD, and to isolate those strategies and features which have been shown to promote effectiveness. To place these findings in context, however, a brief overview will first be presented of the nature and prevalence of CPD, its aims and functions, and the educational approaches adopted in its provision. Influences on the extent and type of CPD programmes offered and on participation in such programmes will also be mentioned, and the numerous and complex methodological issues relevant to the study of the effectiveness of CPD will be discussed.

2 CONTINUING PROFESSIONAL DEVELOPMENT IN CONTEXT

2.1 The history, nature and prevalence of CPD

There is general agreement across the literature about the broad definition and aims of CPD, as given above. At more specific levels, however, agreement is less common and a degree of confusion about the exact nature of CPD is apparent. A large part of this confusion arises from, and is evident in, the use of terminology: CPD developed out of the earlier concepts of continuing professional education (CPE) and continuing medical education (CME). The terms 'education' and 'development' do not refer to exactly the same thing, but the distinction between them is not always reflected in the way they are used, either in the literature or in practice. This has partly resulted from the fact that changes in both the conceptualisation and the practice of on-going professional learning took place before a new term was adopted to take account of the new concepts and practices.

Formal CME provision traditionally emphasised teacher-based, didactic approaches, focusing on clinical topics. But such approaches were criticised and the need for more learner-led approaches and a wider range of topics to be included in CPD became apparent (Singleton and Tylee, 1996; Chambers, 1992). Awareness has also increased of the existing prevalence of self-directed, opportunistic and informal learning among professionals and of the role this has to play in their on-going development: Gear *et al.* (1994), for example, propose that most 'continuous learning' is likely to be initiated, organised, controlled and evaluated by the individual, and that formal inputs play only a supporting role. However, this predilection for self-direction in learning does not in any way imply that doctors do not like to have their learning needs met by formal educational meetings. Indeed, a survey of general practitioners in their first three years of practice shows that (a) they do identify learning needs from their own practice and (b) they choose to meet these needs by short, formal educational meetings (Grant *et al.*, 1998).

In medicine, then, the inadequacy of the existing terms was highlighted by the increasing need for coverage of topics not normally forming part of traditional specialist education, such as management and communication skills training, teamwork and ethics (DOH, 1994). CPD, as a term, reflects all these changes in the provision and perception of professionals' on-going learning, and the practice of CPD within medicine is a development and extension of CPE and CME*. A description of CPD which reflects these changes was given by Todd (1987, p. 5) who suggested that CPD:

> '... makes no preconceptions about whether people learn or are taught, or about the formality of learning activities. People can develop themselves; others can also help them develop; the important thing is that professional development occurs'.

CPD is a relatively new term; however, the implementation of CPE and CME does not itself have a long history. Although the first reported CME course took place in 1935 and there were medical societies, associations and journals which performed a CME function in the 19th century (McKinley, 1990), CME was not discussed as a coherent body of literature until Shepherd's 1960 review

---

*Due to the recent introduction of the term CPD to describe ongoing professional learning, much of the literature refers to CPE or CME and these terms will be used where they appear in original papers.

(Beaudry, 1989) and the first reported conference dedicated to CME did not take place until as late as 1986 (Wilbur, 1987). Having said that, there is still dual use of the terms CME and CPD. For example, the European Union of Medical Specialists still uses the term CME but suggests that this is simply one part of CPD (UEMS, 2008).

In defining CME/CPD, we should also note that there are other strategies which can generate changes in practice, but which are not primarily educational. For example, Allery *et al.* (1997) indicate that organisational factors are effective in inducing change. Other strategies of managing change will also have an effect (Gale and Grant, 1998). Computers may help improve clinician performance (Sullivan and Mitchell, 1995). The classification of clinical guidelines is more problematic. They may be regarded as an assistant to practitioner decisions about appropriate care but might also be most effective when introduced through a specific educational programme, backed up by instrumental reminders to the clinician at the time of consultation (Feder *et al.*, 1997). This review will focus on educational interventions per se but will also address such associated contextual factors.

2.2 The aims and functions of CPD

More than two decades ago, three types of model were described on which CPD programmes might be based (Nowlem, 1988). These still apply. The aims each typically sets out to achieve were set out as follows:

➤ Update models: underpin those programmes which aim simply to communicate or disseminate information. While this is a valid aim, there is a danger with this type of model that the acquisition of information may not be translated into improvements in practice

➤ Competence models: aim to ensure that at least minimum standards for knowledge, skills and attitudes are attained. Programmes based on this type of model may be sufficient to provoke alterations of practice, but they do not necessarily address the issue of whether such alterations lead to optimised patient care outcomes

➤ Performance models: aim not only to help doctors overcome barriers to successful changes in practice, but also to help them resolve clinical concerns. In the medical field, therefore, some emphasis would be placed on healthcare outcomes.

Only a little later, Harden and Laidlaw (1992) offer an approach to CPD which also recognised its integration with practice and placed this in the wider context of the design of learning. Their CRISISS criteria emphasised the following points:

➤ Convenience   makes voluntary participation easy

➤ Relevance   reflects the user's day-to-day role in medical practice

➤ Individualisation   allows learners a say in what is learnt and to adapt the programme to their own needs

➤ Self-assessment   encourages doctors to evaluate their understanding of the subject and to remedy any gaps identified

➤ Interest   arouses attention and encourages learners to participate in the programme

➤ Speculation   recognises controversial and grey areas in medicine

➤ Systematic   offers a planned programme, with coverage of a whole subject or an identified part of it.

Despite the increasing prominence of performance models since the late 1980s, many programmes and authors still do not focus explicitly on aiming to change the outcomes of practice, possibly because they assume that these ought to follow automatically from changes in practice itself. Allery *et al.* (1997), for example, gave changes in doctors' behaviour as one of the important aims of CPD in medicine. Nonetheless, Wilbur (1987), in his report of the first dedicated CME conference, recorded a proposal for CME to occur at, and be relevant to, the workplace, and for programmes to be aimed directly at deficiencies in practice, so that knowledge acquired would be directly relevant to areas of need and therefore more likely to be applied to practice. Abernethy (1990), on the other hand, made direct reference to patient outcomes, stating that:

> 'The whole purpose of continuing medical education is to improve the performance of the doctor in his practice and thus improve the care that patients receive'. (p. 847).

Thus the debates that still occur in the second decade of the 21st century, have been current for many years. What is different now is the involvement of regulation in the area of CPD.

It would seem logical that perceptions of the functions of CPD would reflect its aims, and in some instances this is indeed the case. Parboosingh and Thivierge (1993), for example, stressed the increasing role of CME in the maintenance of professional competence. Not surprisingly, those unclear about the importance of CME attributed to it only a limited purpose, but even when its importance was recognised, it was still not always viewed as having the potential to promote change in professional practice. In some cases, however, CPD was perceived to carry benefits additional to those arising from the achievement of its stated aims. For example, Branthwaite *et al.* (1988) suggested that attendance at CME courses gives general practitioners (GPs) the following opportunities in addition to those for the acquisition of knowledge and the development and maintenance of high professional standards:

➤ Maintenance of interests
➤ Encouragement of an ethos of keeping up-to-date
➤ Stimulation and motivation
➤ Provision of reassurance
➤ Provision of contact and comparison with other GPs
➤ Enhancement of group identity and confidence.

The issue of the confidence that others (patients, the public and managers) have in the doctor is another area in which CPD may serve as an enhancing factor (DoH, 1994). The origins of the regulatory interest in CPD can be traced back to this observation. The Royal Colleges of Physicians (1994) underlined this point:

> 'Given the rapid advances in medical science, the greater expectations of an increasingly informed public and the growing tendency to apportion blame, it is inevitable that we must not only keep abreast of the latest developments, but also that we are seen to do so.'

As well as having stated aims which are wholly worthwhile in their own right, therefore, CPD was also seen as having the potential to fulfil a greater role, both in terms of the development of the individual and of the impressions held of practitioners by others.

And in the UK, a broader context for CPD content arose with the 2001 report into children's heart surgery at Bristol Royal Infirmary (DoH, 2001).

> A major lesson of our Inquiry is that there are a number of non-technical, non-clinical skills of doctors, nurses and managers which are crucially important to the care of patients. We have identified six key areas. They appear to have been relatively neglected in the education and training of healthcare professionals in the past. They must not be in the future. They are:
> ➤ Skills in communicating with patients and with colleagues;
> ➤ Education about the principles and organisation of the NHS, how care is managed, and the skills required for management;
> ➤ The development of teamwork;
> ➤ Shared learning across professional boundaries;
> ➤ Clinical audit and reflective practice; and
> ➤ Leadership.

2.3 Educational approaches, learning and CPD

With increasing calls for the formal documentation and recognition of CPD within medicine, decisions about which activities and approaches to learning should be recognised as acceptable constituents of CPD gained in importance. Along with credit-based systems, which counted the hours spent in certain activities, those activities themselves were judged according to their apparent value, despite lack of evidence.

The criticisms of the traditional approaches used in formal CME programmes have already been mentioned, and Moore's (1995) concerns were representative of the majority of these. He argued that the features of traditional CME:

➤ Are lecture-dominated
➤ Are episodic and non-reinforcing
➤ Involve minimal collaboration between learners and providers
➤ Lack responsiveness to learner needs
➤ Place too much emphasis on the acquisition of credits
➤ Focus too heavily on course production.

In the light of these factors, the principles and features of adult learning, again with no robust evidence base but with a judgment of their appropriateness to a profession, were increasingly being brought into discussions of the nature and provision of CPD (for example, Parboosingh and Thivierge, 1993; Stanley *et al.*, 1993; Stross, 1989; Wilbur, 1987). The following extract from Brookfield (1986, ch. 2) illustrated some of the key features of adult learning theory, much quoted at the time:

> 'Adults learn throughout their lives ... They exhibit diverse learning styles ... and learn in different ways, at different times, for different purposes. As a rule, however, they like their learning activities to be problem-centred and to be meaningful to their life situation, and they want the learning outcomes to have some immediacy of application. The past experience of adults affects their current learning, sometimes serving as an enhancement, sometimes as a hindrance. Effective learning is also linked to the adult's subscription to a self-concept of himself or herself as a learner. Finally, adults exhibit a tendency towards self-directedness in their learning.'

Following Brookfield's view of adult learning, a number of authors propose that self-directed learning, based on experience, should be central to CPD and that formal educational provision, being only a small aspect of lifelong learning, should be complementary to and supportive of this (for example, Rogers, 1997; Gear *et al.*, 1994; Stanley *et al.*, 1993). Picking up the theme of experience-based learning, Cervero (1988) pointed out that professionals' practice is characterised by 'complexities, uncertainties and conflicting values' (p. 85), which is one reason why traditional, didactic approaches to CPD were seen as inadequate – they failed to deal with the specific problems associated with any individual's practice. Nowlem (1988) and Schön (1987) both argued that, due to their in-depth knowledge of the practice setting, peers and colleagues should act as educators, and Schön proposed that they should adopt a coaching-type role: explaining what they would do in any given circumstance and the theoretical framework underlying their proposed choice of action. Much work has been conducted exploring different approaches to experience-based ('experiential') learning and examples of some of these, together with a discussion of their respective strengths and weaknesses and of assessment and validation issues, can be found elsewhere (Stanton and Grant, 1998).

A great deal of discussion has also centred around those concepts of learning as they came into vogue, such as Schön's notion of 'reflection-in-action' (discussed at length by Cervero, 1988) and also around various definitions of elements and stages of learning, such as Houle's Triple Model (1980), which discussed stages of inquiry, instruction and performance. While the majority of these discussions have raised useful theoretical points, it should be noted that most were rhetorical in nature. While the concepts and models they proposed undeniably promoted further discussions of the nature of CPD and the requirements of educational programmes, most have still not yet been adequately tested for their usefulness. Irrespective of the strength of their philosophical and theoretical foundations, their value and thus also their promotion, is not evidence-based.

> As theoretical discussions began to recognise the importance of self-directed and informal learning, the regulatory environment moved towards the measurement of CPD by credits hours and recognised events. This contradiction has continued and now requires resolution.

With respect to the relative importance and popularity of self-directed learning and formal educational activities, a range of each has been cited in the literature and by regulators and professional bodies as constituting acceptable CPD. The following list is drawn from Gear *et al.* (1994), Parboosingh and Thivierge (1993), Stanley *et al.* (1993), Shirriffs (1989) and Stross (1989). The list would be the same, 20 years later but with e-learning replacing audio/videotapes:

Formal activities
➤ Conferences
➤ Courses and educational meetings
➤ Journal clubs
➤ Workshops and small group work.

Self-directed (informal) activities and materials
➤ Journals and texts
➤ Audio/videotapes
➤ Computer-assisted learning
➤ Self-assessment programmes
➤ Teaching
➤ Research
➤ Practice audits

➤ Clinical trainee shops
➤ Discussions with colleagues
➤ Authorship.

Before being hasty about 'effective' learning methods for this group of very high achievers, evidence about individual learning preferences must be taken into account. The UK General Medical Council (2010) endorses this view:

The way in which individual doctors take part in CPD will depend on:
➤ Their specialty
➤ The opportunities available
➤ Their priorities and
➤ Their personal learning styles and preferences.

We encourage this diversity, as without it CPD activities would be less effective.

Considerable variation has been found among doctors regarding which of these learning activities they prefer. For example, Gear *et al.* (1994) found that 10% of their sample preferred formal learning activities and 31% informal ones, but that more than half (55%) preferred a mixture of the two. However, results in this area have not been consistent. Three decades ago, Durno and Gill (1974), for example, found that only 18% of a sample of GPs thought lunchtime meetings to be an acceptable source of regular education (with most, interestingly, considering discussions with hospital doctors their most important source of information and education). Grant *et al.* (1998) also found a high rate of GP attendance at meetings where hospital doctors were the teachers. Both Shirriffs (1989) and Reedy (1979) found traditional, formal activities to be the most popular amongst the doctors they sampled. This is also true of newly-qualified GPs (Grant *et al.*, 1998).

It would appear therefore, that a variety of learning activities and methods can be considered as valid constituents of CPD and that providers of formal programmes have a range of possible options from which to choose. Indeed, Tulinius and Holge-Hazelton (2010) show that mixed learning methods, linked with practice problems are an effective approach.

This view is supported by the Chartered Institute of Personnel and Development (reported in The Mackinnon Partnership, 2007):

> There has been more emphasis on less formal and directive ways in which employees can acquire relevant knowledge and skills. Learning has become more diffuse throughout the organisation and less dependent on a distinct event or activity, such as the training course.

A recent meta-analysis (Bloom, 2005) which looked specifically at the effects of CME on patient care described the complexity of the situation, and underlines that there is not one 'best educational method'. To prescribe or approve learning methods would not be supported by the evidence:

'Burgeoning knowledge from RCTs and meta-analyses of CME is clear on the most effective techniques that alter medical care processes and patient health outcomes – interactive education, audit and feedback, reminders, academic detailing, and other outreach programs, and somewhat less so, clinical practice guidelines and opinion leaders. In addition, combining techniques, for example, interactive education plus academic detailing, leads to even greater effect than either achieves alone. The literature is also clear on the least effective education methods – didactic lectures and distributing printed materials alone. But even a technique of low-efficacy can become useful when combined with interactive tools.'

> Despite many reviews and meta-analyses which show that there is no 'best buy' learning method for CPD, researchers continue to seek this elusive information. It might be better to accept the findings of the many reviews and research projects, and move forward to encompass the many ways in which doctors continue to learn, and build our CME/CPD systems on diversity of practice.

One important point remains to be made. This concerns the call, heard with increasing frequency, for multiprofessional approaches to be taken to the provision of CPD. As yet, despite many years of research, there is minimal evidence for the effectiveness of such approaches.

The rationale for multiprofessional learning is based on the tenet that if different groups work together, they will do so more effectively if they also learn together. Such research as there is suggests that if multiprofessional education is based on real and shared problems, for example, a shared case, and is therefore problem-solving for real, it can be effective. There is no real evidence that learning together in the abstract causes better working together in practice.

The most prominently cited problems of multiprofessional working are:
➤ Differing professional ideologies, terminology, accountability, statutory responsibilities and employment structures
➤ Discrepancies between different professions' perceptions of others' roles and functions, referral patterns and contributions to team work
➤ Different professional knowledge bases, skills, professional roles and self-identities
➤ Diverse professional assumptions about the nature and aims of healthcare, such as, implicitly held healthcare models
➤ Varied professional perceptions of the patient/client/person/the social context and desirable relationships with healthcare professionals
➤ Areas of overlapping knowledge, practice or responsibility
➤ Intra-professional differences.

A relatively recent paper (Tunstall-Pedoe *et al.*, 2003) shows that in an undergraduate interprofessional course:

➤ Students arrive at university with stereotypical views of each other
➤ These views tend to become more exaggerated during the interprofessional course
➤ Students feel that the course would enhance interprofessional working but there are concerns that it forces them to learn irrelevant skills
➤ Students whose parents worked as healthcare professionals held stronger stereotypes than others.

Recent CAIPE* reports show that there is very little evidence about interprofessional learning on which to base either policy or practice. They call for better research. A recent systematic review of interprofessional education (IPE) (Hammick *et al.*, 2008) shows that while this is:

> '... generally well received, enabling knowledge and skills necessary for collaborative working to be learnt; it is less able to positively influence attitudes towards others in the service delivery team. Staff development is a key influence on the effectiveness of IPE and all learners in IPE bring unique values about themselves and others. IPE that reflects the authenticity of practice is more effective. In quality improvement initiatives IPE is frequently used as an effective way of enhancing the practice and improving services.'

Evidence, therefore, remains uncertain. Much more research is required into the experience and effectiveness of multiprofessional interventions before any justification for such a call can be made. It is incontrovertible that different professions must work effectively together. It has not yet been equally demonstrated that learning together is an effective tactic, over and above organisational improvements.

However, the survey of the educational needs of newly qualified GPs (Grant *et al.*, 1998) showed that while multiprofessional education is rejected by the vast majority, the same people endorse being taught by members of other professions in meetings aimed at GPs. So while GPs do not want to learn **with** other professions, they are happy to learn **from** them.

2.4 Influences on CPD provision

Government policy has already been mentioned as one influence on the extent of provision of formal CPD programmes, but other factors also have a bearing on this, as well as on the educational quality of programmes. Two major influences, linked to government policy, are those relating to accreditation and revalidation and to financial input.

---

*Centre for the Advancement of Interprofessional Education. www.caipe.org.uk/resources/

As the Department of Health (1994) pointed out, the (then) CME schemes endorsed by the UK Medical Royal Colleges were all based on systems of credit accumulation, with the achievement of minimum targets over a five-year period. This kind of approach was widespread in medicine across Europe (UEMS, 1994) and was also found farther afield, such as in the MOCOMP* scheme in Canada (Parboosingh and Thivierge, 1993). Fifteen years later, this position is still largely the case. For example, the UK Academy of Medical Royal Colleges has set out their 10 principles of good CPD practice, as follows (Academy of Medical Royal Colleges, 2009):

THE TEN PRINCIPLES FOR COLLEGE/FACULTY CPD SCHEMES

1. An individual's CPD activities should be planned in advance through a personal development plan, and should reflect and be relevant to his or her current and future profile of professional practice and performance. These activities should include continuing professional development outside narrower specialty interests.

2. CPD should include activities both within and outside the employing institution, where there is one, and a balance of learning methods which include a component of active learning. Participants will need to collect evidence to record this process, normally using a structured portfolio cataloguing the different activities. This portfolio will be reviewed as part of appraisal and revalidation.

3. College/Faculty CPD schemes should be available to all members and fellows and, at reasonable cost, to non-members and fellows who practise in a relevant specialty.

4. Normally, credits given by Colleges/Faculties for CPD should be based on one credit equating to one hour of educational activity. The minimum required should be an average of 50 per year. Credits for un-timed activities such as writing, reading and e-learning should be justified by the participant or should be agreed between the provider(s) and College/Faculty directors of CPD.

5. a) Self-accreditation of relevant activities and documented reflective learning should be allowed and encouraged.

   b) Formal approval/accreditation of the quality of educational activities for CPD by Colleges/Faculties should be achieved with minimum bureaucracy and with complete reciprocity between Colleges/Faculties for all approved activities. The approval/accreditation process and criteria should be such as to ensure the quality and likely effectiveness of the activity.

6. Self-accreditation of educational activities will require evidence. This may be produced as a documented reflection. Formal CPD certificates of attendance at meetings will not be a requirement, but evidence of attendance should be provided, as determined by each individual College or Faculty.

---

continued

*Maintenance of Competence

7. Participation in College/Faculty based CPD schemes should normally be confirmed by a regular statement issued to participants which should be based on annually submitted returns, and should be signed off at appraisal.

8. In order to quality assure their CPD system, Colleges/Faculties should fully audit participants' activities on a random basis. Such peer-based audit should verify that claimed activities have been undertaken and are appropriate. Participants will need to collect evidence to enable this process.

9. Until alternative quality assurance processes are established, the proportion of participants involved in random audit each year should be of a size to give confidence that it is representative and effective. This proportion will vary according to the number of participants in a given scheme.

10. Failure to produce sufficient evidence to support claimed credits will result in an individual's annual statement being endorsed accordingly for the year involved and the individual subsequently being subject to audit annually for a defined period. Suspected falsification of evidence for claimed CPD activities will call into question the individual's fitness for revalidation, and may result in referral to the GMC/GDC.

Figure 7: The ten principles for college/faculty CPD schemes

These principles are notable not only because they show that thinking on the credit system has not changed, and that the appropriateness of a variety of learning methods is recognised. What is notable is the new climate of regulation and accountability, and concomitant bureaucracy, into which CPD has been drawn.

A further factor of importance concerns the context of CME/CPD for credit-bearing programmes. In particular, the evidence-based medicine movement has resulted in many such courses. Debates about the validity and value of this approach are not relevant to this review. However, the relevance of evidence, to practice can only be established in the practice context and it will be shown in later sections that objectivity of evidence is nowhere cited as a factor which either facilitates participation in CPD or change in practice, even although a desire to keep up-to-date is important. Taking evidence into ordinary practice as that practice needs, seems to be a main message. The content of CPD should be driven by need rather than externally-referenced factors.

In addition to the issue of quality, questions have also been raised regarding the value of credit accumulation schemes and their actual purpose. Grant (1994) asked why the credit-bearing CME system is in place and what it is designed to achieve:

- deal with bad apples?
- to prove CME is taking place?
- to develop new approaches to CME?
- as a response to a culture of managerialism, accountability and control?

- to ensure that learning opportunities are there?
- to support doctors?

The development of regulatory procedures to deal with poorly performing doctors, has largely nullified the need to deal with the 'bad apple' question by means of CPD. Likewise, 'remedial training' cannot easily be seen as a role for CME/CPD systems.

Despite the continuing prevalence of credit-based systems, it has long been recognised that much actual CPD is not credit-bearing and is likely to remain so. Gear *et al.* (1994) pointed out that much of CPD is difficult for professional bodies to recognise and reward, as it is self-directed and informal in nature. This has now been accepted, and professional bodies are recognising such activity as a relevant part of the CPD process, even although most of this cannot be measured in the form of events: learning in the context of practice is a continuous event best acknowledged through processes rather than events. Likewise, time for reflection on practice and on learning is important and cannot be measured in the same way as attendance at a lecture (Fish and Coles, 1998). All of this does raise the question of what exactly CPD is as well as what credits actually represent, and there is a danger, as Cervero (1988) suggested, that participation in educational programmes may become the primary goal of credit-bearing schemes, rather than learning itself. The fifth principle of the Academy of Medical Royal Colleges recognises this and allows such self-directed or informal learning.

In the light of the difficulties associated with such schemes, Grant (1994) argued that systems based on the accumulation of credits or points may not be the most appropriate. She suggested that locally managed systems based on the developmental needs of particular units and of the doctors working in them (not excluding non-specific or general professional CME) may be more meaningful in terms of ensuring optimal patient care outcomes. In parallel, the Department of Health (1994) proposed that health outcomes should be the criteria against which any investment in CME (in terms of both money and time) should be measured. They acknowledged that there was, as yet, no satisfactory method of doing this.

Perhaps because of this, changes have been modest.

Another way of dealing with the related question of value for money has been put forward by Hollwitz and Danielson (1996), who suggest that financial values and benefits should be assigned to specific interventions, aimed at particular jobs and job functions, in order to foster cost-effective quality assurance. Having said this, however, it must be acknowledged that such types of cost-benefit are only one aspect of the overall professional agenda for learning, albeit an important one, in addressing this issue head-on, Sandars (2010) concludes that:

Measuring the cost-effectiveness of CPD will be a major challenge, since identi-fying the true costs of educational interventions and deciding on the appropriate expected benefits that are relevant to all stakeholders is not easy.

2.5 Influences on participation in CPD programmes

A number of studies have focused on the extent to which doctors and others participate in CPD programmes, with particular emphasis being placed on those factors which motivate or facilitate their participation and on those which deter them or act as barriers. Some motivating and facilitating factors which have been isolated are given in Table 3 below where it can be seen that a general desire to keep up-to-date is the most commonly cited motivator for participation in CPD programmes, and that the opportunity for discussions with colleagues is another common positive influence. These non-instrumental, but highly professional factors must not be lost in future planning. Factors relating to professional competence are also frequently cited. Other influences of note are financial incentives, and satisfaction with programmes attended in the past.

The effects of financial incentives were further investigated by Kelly and Murray (1990) who studied GPs' reasons for attending postgraduate meetings. They found that, while general interest remained a prime motivating factor (cited in 43% of cases), over one-third of attenders (35%) gave monetary incentive as a reason for their participation, while only 29% said that they were motivated by a desire to improve their knowledge. Only 0.4% gave a need to change their practice as a reason for attending. This proportion was half that totalled those who said they did not know why they were there (0.8%)!

More encouragingly, the 1998 survey by Grant *et al.* shows that young doc-tors do reflect on their practice and identify learning needs accordingly.

Making participation in programmes mandatory does not seem to have a great deal of effect on participation rates – Cervero (1988) contended that there are small but insignificant increases only – and the practice has been found to have detrimental effects on participants' satisfaction with the programmes and also on their intentions with respect to future attendance at voluntary courses (Crandall and Cunliff, 1989). Furthermore, Walton (1991) found that changes to practice are considered more satisfying if they are perceived to have arisen from reasons of personal incentive rather than from external pressures. Jones and Fear (1994) found 'overwhelming opposition' to compulsory attendance at CPD programmes by human resources professionals in Wales, although some certification and recognition of CPD activities was welcomed by them.

It seems to be the case, therefore, that the profession maintains a profes-sional view, rather than an instrumental one, of its participation in CPD.

A variety of barriers and deterrents to participation in CPD programmes have also been isolated. For example, differences between trainers and trainees, in terms of their learning styles, have been presented as a possible deterrent,

TABLE 3: Factors which motivate or facilitate participation in CPD

Authors (and dates)	Motivating/Facilitating Factors Isolated
Cividin and Ottoson (1997)	➤ perceived need to confirm or alter current practices ➤ the chance to network with others
Byers et al. (1996)	➤ satisfaction with previous courses/programmes attended
Gear et al. (1994)	➤ the presence of a climate conducive to learning (arising from the Professional Body and prevailing throughout the profession)
DoH (1994)	➤ a need to keep up-to-date ➤ career changes (e.g., of specialty)
Vaughan (1991)	➤ to become/stay up-to-date ➤ to train for new, additional roles ➤ to increase job satisfaction and personal effectiveness
Woolf (1990)	➤ interest in the topics covered (found to be a much stronger motivator than perceived weaknesses)
Fox et al. (1989)	➤ a desire for competence (24%) ➤ pressure to change arising from the clinical environment (14%) ➤ financial incentives (9%)
Wood and Byrne (1980)	➤ a desire among GPs to escape from problems associated with their practices ➤ a desire to communicate with other GPs and other health professionals ➤ a hope for intellectual stimulation ➤ a general desire to keep up-to-date ➤ a need to refresh the memory and increase confidence
Barham and Benseman (1984) and Gross (1976)	➤ working in group settings
Grant et al. (1998)	➤ need identified from practice e.g., management training ➤ peer contact ➤ keeping up-to-date ➤ general interest

although the evidence for this is tentative (Lewis and Bolden, 1989). Other factors, however, are based on more conclusive evidence:

➤ the costs involved in terms of money and time (Langsner, 1994; Wilbur, 1987)

➤ dissatisfaction with the quality of programmes on offer and a lack of personal benefit from participation (Langsner, 1994; Cervero, 1988)

➤ general apathy with respect to education (Cervero, 1988)
➤ a preference for self-directed learning (Cervero, 1988).

Finally, Branthwaite *et al.* (1988) found regular attenders (GPs) at CPD meetings to be more progressive in their work than those who did not attend regularly, to be more concerned about developing their skills and about having the time and scope to practise effectively, and to be more conscientious with respect to developing and improving their work. Commenting on this paper, Gray (1988) raised the question of whether the educational intervention had somehow promoted the development of these characteristics or whether people with such characteristics are those who are more motivated to seek out education.

Gray's question is just one of many which have been raised in connection with the outcomes of CPD, and an in-depth discussion of the findings of outcome studies and of effective educational strategies will follow. There are, however, numerous and complex methodological issues involved in the investigation of the effectiveness of CPD, and as these need to be taken into account if critical appraisal of outcome studies is to be fully informed, they will be dealt with first.

It is these methodological issues which explain the lack of a robust evidence base and might even suggest that there never can be a definitive proven case about the effectiveness of CPD.

3 METHODOLOGICAL ISSUES

Studies investigating the effectiveness of CPD have frequently failed to do so in a conclusive manner (Allery *et al.*, 1997; Ferguson, 1994, Mazmanian *et al.*, 1990) and a commonly cited reason for this lack of conclusiveness is that many such studies rest on weak methodological foundations (Allery *et al.*, 1997; Glazier *et al.*, 1995; Davis *et al.*, 1992). Methodological difficulties have been found in a variety of areas, but are most notable in connection with design issues, with the influence of intervening variables, and with the measurement of outcomes.

The methodological problems identified here are shared by many other areas of education.

3.1 The problem of design

3.1.1. Educational programme design
Problems associated with design fall into two categories: design of educational programmes and design of outcome studies. First, with respect to formal CPD programmes, many of these have been shown to fail to identify the needs of learners and/or their client groups: a problem which often results in the further failure of programme designers to identify and define clear, relevant and measurable objectives (e.g. Allan, 1996; Abernethy, 1990; Bertram and Brooks-Bertram,

1977). One example of the latter problem is provided by a study (which, for obvious reasons, will not be cited) which gave its aim as being to investigate the effectiveness of management training for hospital doctors. The objectives of the educational intervention were presented as: the personal growth and development of participants and an improvement in the extent of their insight into their personal attitudes – not clear, not measurable!

A further problem of programme design in education concerns its description, implementation and replicability. Most forms of education, even e-learning, are to some extent, a function of the personal qualities of the teacher, and the human interaction between teacher and learner. This also means that the qualities of the learners are themselves a factor in the success of any educational intervention. All teachers are different; as are all learners. A seminar or lecture or tutorial or small group session given by one person with one group, will be different from the same planned event given by another teacher with another group.

For research and evaluation, this means that identifying variables, measuring them and then reproducing the behaviour is a very great challenge indeed. Education and learning do not occur in laboratory conditions.

3.1.2 The design of outcome studies

There has never been a satisfactory approach to the outcome of CPD. Almost all reports on the subject conclude with a statement similar to that made by NHS Scotland in 2001:

> 'There is, however, a relative dearth of evaluation of the impact of the changes in performance … to direct patient care.'

In 2002, the Royal College of Nurses concurred.

> '… there is little evidence available on the impact of CPD on patient outcomes.'

The situation had not changed in 2006, when Griscti and Jacono[52] observed that:

> 'Despite a growing body of empirical research on this topic, the effectiveness and impact of continuing education remains underexplored.
>
> Continuing education is intended to ensure healthcare practitioners' knowledge is current, but it is difficult to determine if those who attend these courses are implementing what they have learnt.'

With respect to the design of outcome studies themselves, Allery et al. (1997) raised the following criticisms which still stand:

➤ they frequently fail to use control groups or randomisation
➤ statistical analysis of data is often inadequate
➤ issues of validity are frequently ignored
➤ many studies are correlational and/or retrospective (and are thus unhelpful in terms of increasing the understanding of causal processes).

However, Jacobson *et al.* (1997) in their area argued powerfully that:

> 'The randomised controlled trial alone reflects a reductionist approach that fails to do justice to the philosophy of general practice. The art of medicine is founded on context, anecdote, patient stories of illness and personal experience, and we should continue to blend this with good quality and appropriate research findings in patient care.'

We shall see that such considerations are not irrelevant to educational research in medicine.

Other related criticisms of outcome studies tend to be related to the difficulties inherent in attempting to isolate the influences of particular activities from those of intervening variables and to problems connected with the measurement of outcomes. Both these issues will shortly be discussed in depth but before this, consideration will be given to the randomised controlled study mentioned above. Making reference to the large numbers of participants which are usually involved, Charlton (1996) termed these 'megatrials'. Because of their use of control groups and randomisation techniques, such studies are generally considered to fulfil the requirements of 'good science' (Charlton, 1996) and they are therefore also widely considered to produce findings of guaranteed reliability. However, even this type of study is not immune to criticism. For example, Davis *et al.* (1992), who conducted a review of 50 randomised controlled trials of CME, criticised them on the following grounds:

➤ they give too few details about participants
➤ they give too few qualitative details
➤ they too often use volunteer participants
➤ they too rarely use 'blind' assessment (where assessors are ignorant of the experimental conditions to which individual participants have been assigned).

Charlton has also criticised this type of study, but on the grounds that they involve the deliberate recruitment of large, heterogeneous groups of participants and average findings across these large groups – a practice which he claims is not only of no value, but which can also be dangerously misleading (p. 430)

> 'On formal methodological grounds, an estimate of therapeutic effect derived from a megatrial tells the clinician nothing about the experiences of the individual subjects in that trial: a moderate average improvement may summarise many combinations of benefits, harms and no effect among trial participants.'

Charlton raised these problems with specific reference to drug trials, but his points can nevertheless be applied to the assessment of the effects of educational activities: a moderate average improvement in performance across a large sample of practitioners could (assuming that none suffered a decline in performance as a result of the activity!) have been produced by a combination of a small number of large improvements and a larger number of 'no change' results. Were this to be the case, the findings would say nothing about the reasons for the effectiveness or non-effectiveness of the activity with respect to any individual practitioner's knowledge or performance. A further point, which has been raised by Davis *et al.* and by Charlton, is that randomised controlled trials cannot serve as tests of previously generated hypotheses, but are merely hypothesis-generating exercises themselves, with Charlton describing them as being an example of 'epistemological techniques'.

CPD, as it is currently construed, and as the profession would itself see it, is there to ensure the standards of practice of each individual clinician. It is, by definition, an individual process. Randomised controlled trials are not the best way of evaluating achievement of this intention.

Despite having conducted their review, Davis *et al.* further questioned the validity of making such cross-comparisons because of the inherent variations between trials. Beaudry (1989) also questioned the practice, but for reasons connected with the wide use of non-standardised assessment measures and, in relation to CME programmes, because of the 20 per cent average dropout rate.

A final point raised in connection with large-scale studies is mentioned by Moore (1995), who pointed out that it is generally such large-scale and well-funded studies that manage to demonstrate the success of educational programmes. He argues that studies designed and conducted by the average CME office cannot match the scope of these large-scale studies and that they are therefore unlikely, however well-designed, to be able to replicate their findings.

We are therefore left with findings that are averaged out and so of unknown value in any one case, to those which are also ungeneralisable. This is the perennial problem of educational research.

3.2 The problem of intervening variables

Wergin *et al.* (1988) suggested that as educational activities are not isolated events, they should ideally be considered in relation to contextual influences. This view is reinforced by those studies which have shown that practitioners' behaviour can change as a result of factors which are, or appear to be, unrelated to educational intervention. Walton (1991), for example, found that learning was perceived to be instrumental in doctors' behaviour change in only two-thirds of cases, while Allery *et al.* (1997) found only half of this proportion (i.e. one-third) perceived themselves as having been influenced by educational activity. Taking contextual influences into account is not an easy task, however. As Todd (1987) pointed out, it is extremely difficult to isolate particular interventions or actions as leading to goal achievement, and one of the reasons for this difficulty is the multiplicity of variables which may intervene at various stages of the process. With the expansion of CME into CPD, these problems multiplied, as many of the informal, self-directed activities carried out by learners became even more difficult to isolate in terms of their effects (Gear *et al.*, 1994). The diagram below is presented as an illustration of some of the variables which might intervene in the CPD process, and the points in the process at which they might do this. The challenge presented for research is clear, and this might partially explain the common observation that quality of research in this field is low.[53]

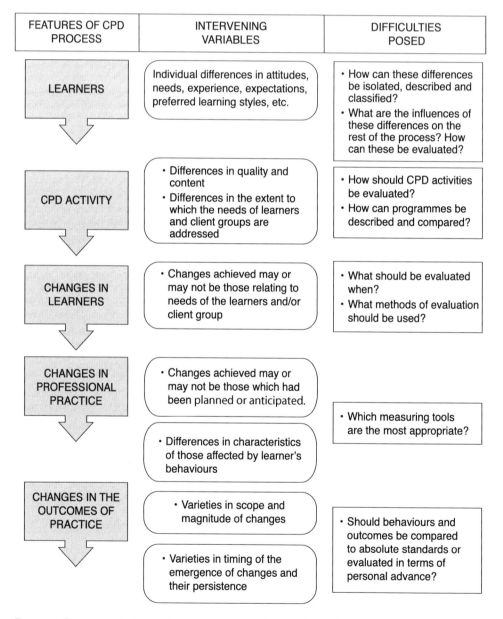

Figure 8: The research difficulties posed by variables which may intervene in the CPD process

While only including a few examples of the huge range of variables that have the potential to intervene at the different stages of the CPD process, this diagram clearly illustrates the complexity, if not the impossibility, of trying to evaluate the influence of an educational activity with respect to professional behaviour or practice outcomes – whether or not the influence of contextual variables is acknowledged by those attempting the evaluation. While it might be possible to establish the causal processes in operation in very general terms, these cannot be predicted for any individual participant, and this circumstance severely impedes the efforts of those attempting to discover the means by which particular changes in practice, or in the outcomes of practice, might best be effected.

3.3 The problem of measurement

The difficulties facing researchers attempting to evaluate the effectiveness of CPD are further compounded by problems associated with the measurement of the outcomes of particular CPD activities. Van der Vleuten (1996) suggests that the area of educational achievement testing is one which is 'in turmoil'. In relation to CPD, this may well still be the case. The extent of the problem was highlighted over 30 years ago by Bertram and Brooks-Bertram (1977) who, having conducted their review of 66 studies of CME outcomes, considered inadequate assessment to be one of the chief reasons for the failure of studies to demonstrate effectiveness in relation to CME programmes. The problems associated with the measurement of outcomes are threefold in nature, and concern, as we have seen:

➤ the type of outcome(s) to be measured
➤ the most appropriate method(s) and tool(s) to use
➤ the timing of the measurement in relation to the timing of the learning.

3.3.1 What should be measured?

One of the main problems with many of the studies which ostensibly concern themselves with the outcomes of CPD, is that the outcomes they choose to study are not connected, or are only very loosely connected, with the aims of CPD, in that they fail to address the issues of changes in practice and in practice outcomes. The literature search conducted for the purpose of this review elicited many studies which involved the measurement of a wide range of such 'outcomes', and these are listed below:

➤ Staff recruitment outcomes
➤ Scores on 'happiness indexes'
➤ Changes in doctors' confidence
➤ Changes in levels of peer support
➤ Changes in the cost of staff training
➤ Further dissemination of knowledge
➤ The intellectual stimulation of programmes
➤ Changes in participants' attitudes, values and beliefs

➤ When and how CME/CPD was used during a period of change
➤ Whether participants' expectations of a programme were met
➤ The extent to which participants had felt challenged by an educational programme
➤ Participants' satisfaction with the type, content and quality of programmes on offer
➤ Whether participants considered the benefits gained from a programme to have been worth the time invested in attending
➤ The types and number of educational meetings attended, and the amount of time expended in attending these.

It would appear that some of the designers of these studies may have fallen into the trap outlined by Dall-Alba and Sandberg (1996, p. 432):

> 'In complex fields of practice, there is a risk that assessment highlights the readily measurable, over-emphasizing detail, rather than promoting essential aspects of competence. In this way, practice is trivialised through assessment which fails to support competence development.'

Others, however, have assessed factors directly related to the aims of CPD. Many studies, for example, have included an increase in practitioner knowledge as an outcome measure (and this might reasonably be presumed to be a prerequisite to changes in practice, even if these do not necessarily follow from it) and the majority have included measures of changes in types of behaviour or level of performance. Some examples of these are listed below:
➤ General clinical management
➤ Use of investigations
➤ Prescribing practices
➤ Counselling strategies
➤ Use of screening techniques
➤ Preventive care practices
➤ Diagnostic accuracy
➤ Referral practices
➤ Follow-up consultations.

It should be noted that practitioners' perceptions of changes in their own performance do not always provide accurate reflections of actual change and that studies investigating changes in practice do not always distinguish between the two (Al-Shehri *et al.*, 1993).

The assessment of patient outcomes is less common than the assessment of doctors' professional performance but, despite this, considerable breadth in the type of indicators selected can be seen in the list of examples from the literature given below:

➤ Safety (in relation to anaesthesia)
➤ Perceptions of care received
➤ Increased coping skills
➤ Emotional well-being
➤ Understanding of conditions experienced
➤ Mortality rates
➤ Increased self-efficacy
➤ Caesarean birth rates.

One point which ought to be raised here is whether, in the light of the factors which researchers consider important to investigate in relation to formal CPD provision, the aims of CPD are sufficiently inclusive. One argument supporting the possibility that they are not, is that a frequent (and perfectly acceptable) outcome of CPD is that doctors take an informed decision **not** to make any change to their practice (Cividin and Ottoson, 1997; Parboosingh and Thivierge, 1993). The general assumption that change in practice is always required and improvement in competence always possible may be ignoring the facts: given the amount of time and effort spent in undergraduate and postgraduate train-ing by all doctors, there are bound to be areas of their practice in which their practices are already up-to-date and in which they are fully competent*. It would be worrying were this not the case. It must be true, therefore, as Fox *et al.* (1989) pointed out, that changes in behaviour are not always necessary, and that some changes which do occur are too small to be measured. Schostak *et al.* (2010)[12] also raise this point from their own research:

> 'The day you stop learning is the day you shouldn't be doing the job', one consul-tant said in an interview. This learning was described as being of two types: either it was learning something new or it was learning that what they were doing was what everybody else was doing and therefore indicative of 'good practice'. This is a form of professional triangulation, that is, a process of comparing experience about similar activities across a range of professional perspectives in order to find what is common, what is different and what is contrasting.

Finally consideration must be given to why some CPD activities do appear to be ineffective. Little published attention has been paid to this, although Davis *et al.* (1995) did put forward some possible explanations for the apparent inef-fectiveness of some activities:
➤ the changes produced are too small to be noted by the methods of assessment used
➤ ceiling effects are operating (such as in the management of hypertension)

---

*Davis *et al.* (1995) proposed a ceiling effect to be generally operating with respect to the management of hypertension, for example.

➤ variations across practitioners, settings and behaviours (caused by multiple intervening variables) lead to the appearance of no effect when results are averaged, as in randomised controlled trials
➤ The methodological problems outlined above will also hamper these efforts.

3.3.2 What methods and tools should be used?

A wide variety of methods and tools of assessment and evaluation have been used in studies of the effectiveness of CPD. In terms of the assessment of patient outcomes, these usually involve one or more of the following: clinical audit techniques, health assessment scales or questionnaires, and occasionally, knowledge quizzes. With respect to professionals' performance, there appear to be at least as many methods and tools of assessment available for assessors to choose from as there are theories of learning. A small selection can include:

checklists	self-assessment tests	peer review
self-report	competence-based methods	chart audits
questionnaires	computer diaries	rating scales
credit accumulation	criterion-referenced methods	
multiple choice tests	learning portfolios	

Each method and type of tool has its own advantages and disadvantages in terms of reliability and validity, generalisability and feasibility (in terms of the time required for evaluation, etc.). Despite these differences, very few studies attempt to compare or even discuss different methods or tools in terms of these characteristics. Reasons for this are related, first, to the difficulty in establishing reliability and validity (which usually involves large numbers of participants and complicated standardisation procedures), and second, to the need to test each participant by means of a variety of time-consuming methods in order for reliability not to be compromised as a result of content specificity problems (the variation displayed by individual learners across different tasks) (Van der Vleuten, 1996).

The advantages and disadvantages of adopting any particular method or tool need to be weighed up within the situational and institutional contexts of the evaluation, with selection depending on the educational environment, the resources available, the attitudes of learners and teacher or trainers, and so on (Norman et al., 1991). In practice, although there are a number of standardised measures available, many evaluations involve the use of non-standardised ones, and these may be specifically designed for particular studies (e.g, French, 1995). However, as Van der Vleuten argues, no single method or tool is a panacea in the assessment of performance, and the content and relevance of tasks to the context of practice and the outcomes to be tapped are more important than the validity of the particular instruments selected for use. What is crucial, he argues, is that those who are being assessed are presented with educationally and professionally valid challenges.

Benett's (1993) point should also be taken into account here, that work-based professional standards are not absolute, but are established, maintained and improved by means of negotiation and professional pragmatism. Therefore, all methods and measures ought to be regularly reviewed (Van der Vleuten, 1996) and the expenditure of a great deal of time and effort on the development of measures may not be appropriate in relation to researching the effects of a CPD intervention. In connection with this issue, Van der Vleuten has also contested the current popularity of objective measures and the fact that many now consider them to be, by definition, superior to more subjective measurement techniques (Van der Vleuten *et al.*, 1991). This stance is contested on two grounds: first, on the basis that objective measurement methods do not necessarily produce more reliable results than subjective ones; and second, on the basis that reproducibility of findings is a more useful goal of measurement than objectivity *per se*, and that the influence of subjective error on reproducibility is limited. The use of subjective measures also removes the need for large-scale validation and standardisation studies.

These issues of assessment suggest that perhaps this is not the best way to judge whether CPD has been effective. It would be difficult to find one assessment system that measured the effects of CPD, and not feasible to assess each doctor individually in relation to the learning undertaken.

3.3.3 When should effectiveness of CPD be evaluated?

The timing of the evaluation of the outcomes of CPD activities in relation to the timing of those activities is something which has not received a great deal of attention in the literature, but is an issue in need of some consideration. As Gibbs *et al.* (1994) found, perceptions of the value of educational experience change over time: the 'feel good' factor has a tendency to decrease on participants' return to work where the benefits of newly acquired knowledge and skills may not be immediately apparent. Boud (1988) suggested that an initial evaluation may need to include the identity and exploration of feelings engendered by the experience of the CPD activity so that these cannot then bias later evaluations. Al-Shehri *et al.* (1993) proposed that indications of the feature(s) of an activity participants later find useful in practice can be addressed within a reasonable period, after the activity has taken place – unfortunately they do not specify what constitutes a reasonable period. The sparseness of information in this area suggests a need for further research into the timing and persistence of the outcomes of CPD activities in relation to the timing of the activities themselves. Perhaps different CPD types might require different time-lapses for their proper evaluation.

Taking all these methodological issues together, it can clearly be seen that the evaluation of the effectiveness of CPD is a far from simple task and that there are many difficulties and complexities facing the researcher in this field. This background of confused definitions and aims as well as unpredictable outcomes, widely varying methods and tools of assessment must be kept in mind during any consideration of the findings of the outcome studies in this field.

4 FINDINGS OF THE REVIEW

For the purpose of the 2000 review on which this updated version is based, the following databases were searched for journal articles published from 1990 onwards:

➤ BIDS (Bath Information and Data Service), Social Science Citation Index
➤ Medline
➤ First Search
➤ ERIC (Educational Resources and Information Centre), Current Index of Journals in Education.

Keywords used included: continuing medical education; continuing professional development; nurse education; health professional education; evaluation; outcome measures.

In total, 2561 articles were found in connection with CME and CPD, but of these only 118 remained when 'outcome' was added as a search item. Sixty-two of these 118 papers reported studies in connection with the medical profession, 36 to nursing and allied professions (e.g, health visiting) and 20 to other professions. The criteria for studies to be included in this report were that the outcomes they assessed were in connection with patient care, practitioner knowledge or practitioner behaviour/performance. As reported earlier, few studies which purport to investigate the outcomes of CPD address themselves directly to the attainment of its aims and this was reflected by the result of applying these criteria to the 118 outcome studies elicited by the search: only 16 remained for consideration. Of these 16 studies, six involved doctors, six nurses or members of allied professions, one both doctors and nurses and one was multidisciplinary. Only one study did not concern healthcare practitioners and that involved college staff. Thirteen studies considered practitioner outcomes alone, one considered patient outcomes alone, and two considered both. It must be remembered that the references cited do include two review articles by Davis *et al.* (1992; 1995).

In 2011, further papers were added, including two literature reviews (Schostak *et al.*, 2010; The Mackinnon Partnership, 2007). No new conclusions were reached. The literature since 2000 has not changed the picture, with the possible exception of the continuing rise of regulation.

4.1 The extent to which CPD aims were achieved

The literature mainly offers evidence (as opposed to discussion) about formal CME/CPD events rather than about on-going practice-based, individual CPD based on reflection and experience. The following review of evidence must be interpreted in this light, and should not be seen as promoting that view of CPD. The effects of creating and managing learning opportunities within everyday professional life have not been addressed in the research literature: learning from patients, case discussions, referral letters, effects of the management of patients, in-practice reviews, discussion with colleagues. It is important to recognise these ways of continuing to learn and refine them, making them more conscious and purposeful as the basis of a professional's approach to life-long learning. However, the literature is inadequate in addressing these less perceptible and less measurable methods.

4.1.1 Results in connection with patient outcomes

Three studies which reported practitioners' use of activities aimed at patient outcomes found improvements to have occurred as a result of those activities. In the first of these studies, patients with breast cancer who were cared for by nurses who had undergone a training programme on the subject reported more positive perceptions of the care they received than did a control group and they also displayed a greater level of knowledge about their condition and lower anxiety levels (Alexander, 1990). The differences were found to be statistically significant in each case. Gerrard *et al.* (1993) found that training health visitors in the detection, treatment and prevention of postnatal depression had a positive influence on the emotional well-being of their clients.

The third study showing improvements in patient outcomes (Malenka and O'Connor, 1995) reported the effects of a collaborative study group which aimed to improve patient care by monitoring the outcomes of coronary artery by-pass graft (CABG) operations across institutions in northern New England. The group met at least three times a year and operated in the following ways:

➤ information was disseminated by newsletter to all members of the group between meetings

➤ all members were trained in the use of quality improvement tools and techniques

➤ members conducted a comparative process analysis in order to learn about best practices.

The study found that average in-hospital mortality in relation to CABG had decreased significantly in the three years since the group had been established. The group had also discovered the most common cause of death following CABG across the hospitals in the region and a further study was being conducted to try to discover why this problem was occurring and what improvements could be made to patient care to reduce its incidence and/or lessen the severity of its consequences. What is notable about this intervention is its basis in real practice.

4.1.2 Results in connection with practitioner outcomes

Thirteen of 15 studies reviewed concerned with practitioner outcomes claimed to have achieved positive changes in knowledge, behaviour and/or performance, with the findings of the other two being inconclusive. Statistical analysis of findings was not possible or appropriate in all cases, but significance was claimed in four studies (Hadiyono *et al.*, 1996; Mann *et al.*, 1996; Alexander, 1990; Fleming *et al.*, 1990). Change had been found in relation to a wide range of topics and behaviours, as can be seen from the list presented below:

- Collaborative care and multidisciplinary working
- Prescription practices
- Knowledge and practices relating to pain management
- Knowledge of health promotion issues
- Practitioners' health-related behaviour
- Expansion of practitioners' professional roles
- The 'timely application' of theory to practice
- Diagnostic accuracy (two studies)
- Referral practices
- Changes to teaching strategies and curriculum planning
- The detection, treatment and prevention of postnatal depression
- Knowledge relating to gerontology
- Knowledge and practices relating to cardiac arrhythmias
- Knowledge and practices relating to breast cancer nursing

Four studies were found to have achieved particularly interesting findings and these will therefore be discussed in more detail. Two of these (Mann *et al.*, 1996; Crandall, 1990) raised issues connected with variations in outcome across participants and the need for contextual factors to be considered in connection with outcomes.

Mann *et al.*'s paper reports the outcomes of a problem-based training programme concerned with the promotion of cardiac health. The programme involved practitioners based at three different worksites and coming from a variety of professions related to healthcare (including doctors, nurses, dieticians, pharmacists and social workers). The goals of the study were: to promote collaborative care and multidisciplinary working, to increase up-to-date and specific knowledge, to increase awareness of available resources, and to increase practitioners' skills with respect to changing other people's behaviour. All goals were met in all sites, but there were clear variations in the extent to which change took place, or was perceived to have taken place, across the three sites (for example, to the extent to which inter-disciplinary collaboration was fostered) and between disciplines (for example, in all areas except community development and health promotion, physicians were the least likely professional group to perceive that they had learned anything). These differences raise the question of the context in which training takes place. Given the interdisciplinary nature of this programme it is likely that most participants would be relatively uninformed at the outset in relation to some areas about which information was presented. In such circumstances, the level at which the information would need to be pitched would probably not be sufficiently high for physicians to gain very much except in those areas with which they would not themselves be very familiar, and these were likely to have been fewer in number than those with which the members of other professions were unfamiliar.

Crandall's study (1990) was based on a qualitative case study approach and followed the practice of five doctors over a period of six months after they had attended a one-day conference on cardiac arrhythmias. Although the conference organisers had aimed to promote changes in practice, this objective had not been made explicit to those attending the conference. Three of the five doctors studied committed themselves, on the day of the conference, to making changes to their practice, while a fourth later made a decision to do so. Of the nine changes the doctors had committed themselves to making, six were still being practised six months later. However, the differences between the participants, in terms of both decisions to change practice and actual changes made, prompted Crandall to state that:

> 'CME does make a difference, but program planners must pay attention to the circumstances under which it does' (p. 346).

Dalton's (1996) study highlighted the importance of the timing of evaluations of the effectiveness of CPD activities and the need for gains in participants' knowledge to be followed up so that any consequent changes in practice might be observed. The study concerned the results of an educational programme which was designed to increase nurses' knowledge in connection with pain management and which anticipated that increases in knowledge would lead to changes in practice. The programme did not significantly increase the knowledge of the participating nurses but, despite this, changes in practice which were attributed to the programme were seen to emerge about six months after its completion. These changes involved increased documentation (e.g., of pain intensity ratings and anxiety levels) and improved prescribing practices. This study shows that the evaluation of the effectiveness of CPD activities needs, therefore, to be carefully conducted in order to assess the magnitude and scope of their effects – as this study has shown, small initial changes may have consequences beyond those which might have been expected. Further research is required into the timespan over which the consequences of particular activities may become apparent, together with any contextual influences on this.

The fourth study of particular interest was that of De Buda and Woolf (1990). The intervention outlined in this paper ('Saturday at the University') was a series of single-day events for family physicians which covered three Saturdays in the spring and another three in the autumn of three consecutive years. The paper reports on the effectiveness of the programme as judged at the end of the first year. The reason this study is of interest is that it demonstrates that formal educational programmes aimed at large numbers of participants, are not necessarily ineffective (despite the extent of the criticism which has been directed towards them). Each of the 'Saturday at the University' training days used the same format, involving a series of 10-minute presentations, each of which was followed by 10 minutes of questions (some written and some from 'the floor'). Each major topic covered, involved a series of presentations by the same person and each presentation focused on just three main points, which were reinforced by hand-outs. Participants were also given paper copies of all slides used in presentations. Evaluation of the outcomes of this programme was by means of a self-report postal questionnaire sent out to doctors three months after they had attended the last of the six days which comprised the first year of the course. Ninety-three per cent of respondents said that they had gained in knowledge and that they were applying their new knowledge to the care and management of their patients. Possibly because the findings were based on self-reports, De Buda and Woolf were quite tentative in claiming the effectiveness of the programme, concluding (p. 283):

> 'There is evidence that a single CME activity might not result in change (Fox *et al.*, 1989) but may help to prepare for change, and it is likely that this was achieved by "Saturday at the University".'

The authors did, however, put forward several suggestions for the apparent success of this programme and these will be discussed in the next part of this paper, together with other factors which have emerged, both from this report and from earlier studies, as enhancing the effectiveness of the CPD process. What emerges is not a straightforward picture.

The findings of these studies underline the influence of contextual and intervening variables and the problems associated with trying to isolate their effects from those of CPD activities.

4.2 Influences on the effectiveness of the CPD process

Several of those whose work has been reviewed here have proffered suggestions as to the reasons underlying the relative success of their programmes, and these are given in Table 4:

TABLE 4: Education providers' perceptions of the reasons for their success

Authors (and dates)	Suggestions Made
Hadiyono *et al.* (1996)	➤ That examples of good practice are established as normative behaviour amongst groups of colleagues
Kushnir *et al.* (1996)	➤ That speakers at formal presentations be expert in the field they are discussing

continued

Malinka and O'Connor (1995)	➤ That a person of authority be in charge of educational programmes ➤ That, where cross-institutional collaboration is required, one person at each institution be responsible for the management of the intervention
Alexander (1990)	➤ That evaluation of the effectiveness of activities is an essential part of programme development ➤ That the evaluation of patient outcomes, while challenging, is an integral part of programme evaluation
De Buda and Woolf (1990)	➤ That the development of good interpersonal relationships between participants be promoted

The importance of the accurate assessment of need was raised in nearly all of the studies reviewed, and many propose it as being the crucial first step in the planning of effective CPD activities (e.g., Citivin and Ottoson, 1997; Allan, 1996; Van der Vleuten, 1996; De Buda and Woolf, 1990). This topic therefore warrants further discussion. Another area which will be discussed in some depth is concerned with those strategies and features which have been shown to enhance effectiveness across a range of different types of intervention.

4.2.1 The Importance of needs assessment

Laxdal (1982) and Davis and Thomson (1996) described learning needs in terms of gaps between ideal and actual practitioner performance, but others expanded on this and argued that the needs of practitioners' client groups should also be taken into account when CPD activities are planned (e.g., Alexander, 1990). It also seems logical that any deficiencies in terms of knowledge and understanding will need to be identified and rectified if such gaps are to be filled. Davis and Thomson propose that effective needs assessment can promote the targeting of activities to the areas of need and the removal of barriers to change in the practice setting.

Laxdal suggests that, although needs assessment is vital, it is poorly understood and difficult to do well, and that it is therefore often inadequately carried out. This view was supported by the findings of Williams et al. (1989) who discovered that the usual method of analysis performed in relation to a standard needs assessment survey instrument (in terms of frequency counts and average scores for expressed preferences) would have led, if acted upon, to a series of courses heavily biased towards only one or two topics which would have disappointed more than half of those who had completed the survey. They found that factor analysis provided a more realistic picture. However, factor analysis is a difficult statistical technique and interpretation can be quite challenging, and many would be deterred from attempting it on these grounds.

One suggestion that has been raised in the literature is that practitioners should conduct their own needs assessment, possibly with the help of computerised diary packages (Parboosingh and Thivierge, 1993), but others have questioned the reliability of this method. Davis and Thomson (1996), for example, ask whether doctors are really able to judge their own competencies, and Chambers (1992) argues that, in its extreme form, self-identification of learning needs:

> '.... puts the onus on practitioners to solve the deep-rooted and vexed questions surrounding the relationships between theory and practice, subject knowledge and competence in these fields — thus absolving educators themselves of the need to continue to address such issues.' (p. 16).

A possible solution which has been proposed to this problem is the use of the Delphi technique (Dunn and Hamilton, 1985). As Chambers explains, this technique involves the setting up of a consensus regarding the competencies needed by members of a profession by a group of around 20 expert practitioners of that profession. Although the technique produces only a very general assessment of needs, the criteria, once established, can be used in the form of a questionnaire to help learners identify their own individual needs. Chambers does point out, however, that learners do not rate themselves as well as their educators do and that caution is therefore required. Tracey et al. (1997) have also demonstrated the inaccuracy of GPs' self-assessments of knowledge. So, even this essential element is not without its challenges.

Despite the heavy emphasis placed by authors on the importance of accurate needs assessment, few viable suggestions have been found with respect to how such accuracy might be achieved. The point made by the Department of Health in 1994 clearly still applies almost 20 years later: there is a need for practical, effective and acceptable methods by which the learning needs of individual doctors can be objectively determined. At this time, techniques such as audit, critical incident review, 360° assessment, patient feedback and appraisal try to fill this requirement. However, the effectiveness and accuracy of these methods remains largely without research.

Having recognised the importance of needs assessment, one further factor must be considered: the question of whose needs? Learning or development needs will be assessed in the context of the practice and of quality of service to patients and the community. There are many formal ways of involving patients in such a needs assessment (e.g., Wiles, 1996). There are also models of needs assessment in primary care which are rooted in the consultation and have a patient orientation. The Canadian MOCOMP programme (Parboosingh and Thivierge, 1993) was such a model. There are others, often less well-known and well-evaluated. These include experiential learning, service-based learning, personal learning plans, learning contracts, portfolio-based learning, PUNs and

DENs, self-assessment, appraisal, peer-assessment and tutoring and competence-based assessment. These, and others, are discussed in Stanton and Grant (1997).

It should also be remembered that, given unreliability, limited scope and frequent lack of practical feasibility of formal methods, needs assessment can be relatively informal, based on professional judgment and organisational development, and be still just as effective. Grant *et al.* (1998) have shown this, as have Fish and Coles (1998).

4.2.2 Effective strategies and features of CPD activities

Davis and Thomson (1996) present a list of strategies in terms of the apparent extent of their effectiveness in producing positive changes in performance:

Highly effective strategies:	➤ practice-linked strategies ➤ multifaceted strategies (especially those including three or more elements) ➤ academic outreach e.g. promotion of rational prescribing behaviour by specially trained academics
Moderately effective strategies:	➤ audit/feedback (especially if individualised and presented by a person of authority) ➤ opinion leaders
Ineffective strategies:	➤ educational materials (especially unsolicited, printed material sent via the mail) ➤ formal CME (especially didactic courses)

The last strategy, however, should not include rejection of short educational meetings with both didactic and interactive components (Grant *et al.*, 1998). Likewise, this list may well be tempered in practice by individual and contextual factors.

Moore (1995) has claimed the changes that occurred in the healthcare environment resulted in positive approaches in CPD, such as an increased emphasis on learning and learning activities with direct relevance to clinical practice, the integration of CPD into the healthcare system, and an increase in co-operative planning of activities. An increased focus on research-based evidence regarding those features and strategies with a positive influence on the CPD process, rather than on the on-going (and apparently self-perpetuating) rhetoric which is evident in much of the literature, is one way in which these changes in approach can be fostered and promoted.

Davis and Thomson are strongly supportive of self-directed learning in preference to more formal activities, and give the following as their reason (p.162):

> 'There is already evidence that physicians exposed to self-directed learning, often co-ordinated through small-group, problem-based strategies continue their practice of self-directed learning, keeping up-to-date later in practice.'

What is cause and correlation, however, is not clear. But, Tracey *et al.*'s (1997) findings do call into question the whole basis of self-directed learning and suggest that not all formal activities are ineffective, as the study by de Buda and Woolf has demonstrated. A consideration of those features of activities which serve to enhance the effectiveness of both formal and self-directed activities may be more productive than a rigid endorsement of one type of activity over another.

The 1992, 1995 and 1998 reviews by Davis *et al.*, and Davis and Thomson's (1996) paper all point to the following features as being those which can enhance effectiveness.

a) Predisposing features	those which predispose individuals to change (e.g., those which impart information)
b) Enabling features	those which enable the change by facilitating its application in the practice environment (such as the rehearsal of desirable behaviours)
c) Reinforcing features	those which reinforce the change (e.g., reminders and feedback)

The influence of these features is further supported by the strong resemblance they bear to those incorporated into the PRECEDE-PROCEED model of behaviour change (Green *et al.*, 1980; Green and Kreuter, 1991) which has been shown to be effective in relation to health promotion. In their 1992 review, Davis *et al.* found that while activities incorporating predisposing features alone were moderately successful in terms of achieving improvements in performance, they were almost always ineffective with respect to improving patient outcomes. Where either enhancing or reinforcing features, or both, were combined with predisposing features, however, the effectiveness of the activities concerned was greatly enhanced.

> Davis *et al.* concluded, therefore, that the most important positive influence on the CPD process was the use of *practice-based, enabling and reinforcing strategies in conjunction with predisposing strategies and adequate needs assessment.* At this point, it becomes clear that effective CPD must be seen as a process rather than an educational event.

Eraut (2001) also concluded that a similar model would be effective for CPD, using stages of identification of learning needs, prioritisation of those needs and then matching learning opportunities and activities to them.

This, perhaps daunting, conclusion was endorsed by the 1995 review and has also been supported by Ottoson (1995) who incorporated the three types of features into her 'Application Process Framework' – a theoretical model of the stages involved in designing and planning a CPD programme. Schostak *et al.*'s (2010) review also supports this approach:

> 'The evidence in the literature indicated that successful learning was much more likely to occur through active modes of learning than through passive ones. This typically involved linking CPD with needs analysis assessments and the development of multiple learning activities. Furthermore, CPD was described as being at the heart of knowledge translation, bridging the transitions from theory to practice. Another recurrent theme, centred upon minimising the gap between theory and practice, was the principle of ensuring that knowledge does not remain abstract, i.e. as something that is learnt outside the practice arena. Thus, the literature recommended that effective knowledge should be integrated with everyday working practices, and combined with follow-up activities in order to ensure reinforcement and critical development.'

Mazmanian (2002) also recognises that needs assessment is a precursor to change and that CPD activity can be wide and varied. This leads him to question the credit-based system and to assert that:

> ... CME must be self-directed by the physician, including management of the content and context for learning.

Ottoson (1995) also stressed the importance of the context in which the elements of the programme were received by participants. Grilli and Lomas (1994) have pointed out that innovations are adopted faster if they:

➤ Represent only small departures from current practices
➤ Are not unduly complex
➤ Can be tried out in practice
➤ Are compatible with current thinking.

Gale and Grant's (1997) research into the management of change in medicine supports these findings. They show acceptance that there is a problem, recognition of the solution and support for the change are crucial. In addition, presenting the change as incremental and enabling demonstration of the change are also powerful tools.

The successful programme designed by De Buda and Woolf, while displaying features common to traditional, and often unsuccessful CME interventions (such as large numbers of participants and didactic presentations) can also be seen to display examples of those features described by Davis *et al.* as being characteristic of effective activities. First, the designers conducted a needs assessment in relation to the programme while it was still at the planning stage. Second, by limiting presentations to 10 minutes each, and by varying the type and pace of input by introduction of 10 minutes of questions between each presentation and the next, participants' attention to the predisposing elements of the course was enhanced, as was the likelihood of their retaining the information presented. The likelihood of the retention of information was further enhanced by the restriction placed on presentations to emphasise no more than three key points, salient to practice. The amount of time which was devoted to dealing with participants' questions (up to 200 were dealt with per day) could be considered an enhancing feature, and the programme hand-outs and notes served as reinforcing features as participants reported having used them when needed in consultations with patients.

This consideration of De Buda and Woolf's programme in terms of those features proposed as enhancers of the effectiveness of the CPD process, has rendered its success easily interpretable, and the importance of the features concerned has again been underlined. An inspection of the suggestions made by the other providers of activities in the studies reviewed here further supports the role of strategies which incorporate enabling and reinforcing features, as most of those described as possible enhancers of effectiveness could be described as one or other of these.

It is important to note here, then, that a practice-based and learner-orientated system of CME/CPD does not imply that the entire process should occur in the practice, nor that it should not contain a didactic element.

5 SUMMARY OF IMPORTANT ISSUES

The literature review has given rise to some important points which might be used for policy planning. They are reiterated here:

➤ Awareness has increased of the prevalence of self-directed learning among professionals and of the role this has to play in their on-going development: most 'continuing learning' is likely to be initiated, organised, controlled and evaluated by the individual, and formal inputs play only a supporting, albeit important, role

➤ It is important to note that self-directed learning implies only that the learners are in a position to decide what needs they have (deriving from their own, or their organisation's needs) and to play a major part in deciding what benefit has been derived from the CPD undertaken. That CPD, however, can take any acceptable and relevant form ranging from relatively traditional and formal to highly innovative and informal methods. Teaching and learning method is not the key variable.

Three models of CME/CPD are commonly seen:

➤ *'Update models'* aim simply to communicate or disseminate information. There is a danger with this type of model that the acquisition of information may not be translated into improvements in practice

➤ *'Competence models'* aim to ensure that at least minimum standards for knowledge, skills, and attitudes are attained. Programmes based on this type of model may be sufficient to provoke alterations of practice, but they do not necessarily address the issue of whether such alterations lead to optimised patient care outcomes

➤ *'Performance models'* (which are beginning to gain prominence) aim not only to help doctors overcome barriers to successful changes in practice, but also to help them resolve clinical concerns

➤ The objective measurement of the outcome of CPD is usually too fraught with confounding variables and practical problems to be undertaken. However, demonstration of the benefit of CPD, building on professional judgement is feasible and meaningful

➤ Evidence suggests that individual doctors vary considerably in their preference for different learning methods. These preferences must be taken into account rather than adopting a rigid view of how doctors 'ought' to like to learn. Evidence suggests that learning method is less important than many other factors

➤ While credit-bearing CPD schemes have increased the number and variety of programmes on offer to doctors, they have not always guaranteed their quality, relevance or effect

➤ In addition to the issue of quality, questions have also been raised regarding the value of credit accumulation schemes on the grounds that they do not directly address the issue of patient care outcomes. This raises the question of what exactly CPD is, as well as what credits actually represent. There is a danger that participation in educational programmes may become the primary goal of credit-bearing schemes, rather than learning itself

➤ In the light of the difficulties associated with credit-based schemes, systems based on the accumulation of credits or points may not be the most appropriate. Locally managed systems based on the development needs of particular units and of the doctors working in them may be more meaningful in terms of ensuring optimal patient care outcomes

➤ Much actual CPD is not credit-bearing and is likely to remain so. This is difficult for professional bodies to recognise and reward, as it is self-directed and informal in nature. Attempts should be made to further increase the recognition of such learning

➤ Questions of value-for-money cannot be avoided. Although there are no satisfactory ways of doing this, a broad framework of responsibility should be established which is likely to increase cost-effectiveness. This will involve allocating responsibility for ensuring that the necessary resources are available; for setting standards; for contributing towards costs and demonstrating commitment to CPD

➤ Value for money will be increased when CPD planning integrates both personal needs and interests with the development plans of organisations

➤ Changes to practice are considered more satisfying if they are perceived to have arisen from reasons of personal incentive rather than from external pressures.

➤ Many formal CPD programmes fail to identify the needs of learners and/or their client groups, although it could be argued that responsibility for needs assessment is the learner's who then chooses what provision to accept

➤ The huge range of variables which have the potential to intervene at the different stages of the CPD process illustrates the complexity, if not the impossibility, of trying to evaluate the influence of an educational activity on professional behaviour or practice outcomes – whether or not the influence of contextual variables is acknowledged by those attempting the evaluation. While it might be possible to establish the causal or correlational processes in operation in very general terms, these cannot be predicted for any individual participant, and this circumstance severely impedes the efforts of those attempting to discover the means by which particular changes in practice, or in the outcomes of practice, might best be effected

➤ In complex fields of practice, there is a risk that assessment highlights the readily measurable, over-emphasising detail rather than promoting essential aspects of competence. In this way, practice is trivialised through assessment which fails to support professional development

➤ The general assumption that change in practice is always required and improvement in competence always possible, may be ignoring the facts: given the amount of time and effort spent in undergraduate and postgraduate training by all doctors, there are bound to be vast areas of their practice which they are already up-to-date and in which they are fully competent. CPD might simply demonstrate this fact

➤ Work-based professional standards are not absolute, but are established, maintained and improved by means of negotiation and professional pragmatism

➤ The timing of assessment of the outcomes of CPD activities in relation to the timing of the activities themselves is something which has not received a great deal of attention in the literature, but which is an issue in need of some consideration

➤ CPD does make a difference, but programme planners must pay attention to the circumstances under which it does. These may include:
  - *predisposing features*: those which predispose individuals to change (e.g. those which impart information)
  - *enabling features*: those which enable the change by facilitating its application in the practice environment (such as the rehearsal of desirable behaviours)
  - *reinforcing features*: those which reinforce the change (e.g. reminders and feedback)
  - *assessment of the needs* of practitioners and their clients/patients.
  - consideration of the *influence of relevant contextual* factors.

➤ There is a need for practical, effective and acceptable methods by which the learning needs of individual doctors can be determined. Although needs assessment is vital, it is poorly understood and difficult to do well, and it is often inadequately carried out. Given the unreliability, limited scope and frequent lack of practical feasibility of formal methods, needs assessment can be relatively informal, based on professional judgment and organisational development, and still be just as effective

➤ Innovations are adopted faster if they represent only small departures from current practices, if they are not unduly complex, if they can be tried out in practice and if they are compatible with current thinking

➤ An increased focus on research-based evidence regarding those features and strategies with a positive influence on the CPD process, rather than on the on-going (and apparently self-perpetuating) rhetoric about learning theories and methods which is evident in much of the literature, is one way that changes in approach can be fostered and promoted. As yet, there is minimal evidence for the effectiveness of some widely advocated approaches.

> Our conclusion must be that the effectiveness of CPD is a function of the process and the context in which it occurs and not a function of one or another specific event, educational intervention or accumulated hours of continuing education in a professional life.

6 MOVING ON FROM HERE: A FOCUS ON PROCESS

This review has shown that there is no educational panacea, no 'most effective' learning method, and no 'best buy' outcome measures. It has also shown there is a more productive way of looking at the question of outcomes than seeking specific events and observable consequences; that a more productive way involves looking at how the conditions for effectiveness of CPD activity (of whatever type) can be created. And that is by establishing a process and culture rather than specifying particular events, educational experiences or types of education or certain outcomes. It might be best to base conclusions about the outcomes of CPD on professional judgement, explicitly made and defended.

We must therefore focus on improving the quality of the process and making it more relevant to individual needs and interests, service-needs, the needs of the team and the practice. The process of planning and undertaking CPD must be managed so that those needs and interests are met, and outcomes can be judged in practical and professionally appropriate ways. CPD will therefore be a positive contribution to development. Different processes are used to identify and deal with poor performance – that cannot be a function of CPD.

In terms of development work, it can be proposed that:

➤ A wide range of acceptable and feasible approaches to needs assessment and CPD planning for the individual and the unit be developed and existing ones described, and supporting documentation provided

➤ A wide range of appropriate methods of education or development be described

> ➤ Practical and professionally relevant guidelines for the reasonable evaluation of outcomes be prepared, based on professionally appropriate methods and explicit professional judgment.

Practices and practitioners demonstrating CME/CPD management processes, by implementing at least one of the suggested approaches from each stage, should receive due recognition and reward.

> Available evidence all suggests that CPD should be developed as a process of planning, doing, and reviewing effect. Focusing on the nature and management of that process will be the most effective strategy.

REVIEW REFERENCES

Abbott L, Dallat J, Robinson A. Videoconferencing in continuing education: An evaluation of its application to professional development at the University of Ulster (1990–5). *Educational Media International.* 1995; **32**(2): 77–82.

Abernethy RD. Continuing Medical Education for general practitioners in North Devon. *Postgrad Med J.* 1990; **66**: 847–8.

Academy of Medical Royal Colleges Continuing Professional Development. Guidelines for Recommended headings under which to describe a College or Faculty CPD scheme; 2009. www.rcgp.org.uk/PDF/ACADEMY%20GUIDANCE%20CPD%20HEADINGS.pdf

Alexander MA. Evaluation of a training program in breast cancer nursing. *J Contin Educ Nurs.* 1990; **21**(6): 260–6.

Allan J. Learning outcomes in higher education. *Stud High Educ.* 1996; **21**: 93–108.

Allery L, Owen P, Hayes T, *et al.* Differences in continuing Medical Education activities and attitudes between trainers and trainees in general practice. *Postgrad Educ Gen Pract.* 1991; **2**: 176–82.

Allery LA, Owen PA, Robling MR. Why general practitioners and consultants change their clinical practice: a critical incident study. *BMJ.* 1997; **314**: 870–4.

Al-Shehri A, Bligh J, Stanley I. A draft charter for general practice continuing education. *Postgrad Educ Gen Pract.* 1993; **4**: 161–7.

Amesberger G. Evaluation of experiential learning programmes: qualitative and quantitative approaches. *Journal of Adventure Education and Outdoor Leadership.* 1996; **13**(2): 58–62.

Bachman JA, Kitchens EK, Halley SS, *et al.* Assessment of learning needs of nurse educators: continuing education implications. *J Contin Educ Nurs.* 1992; **23**(1): 29–33.

Barham PM, Benseman J. Participation in continuing Medical Education of general practitioners in New Zealand. *J Med Educ.* 1984; **59**: 649–54.

Beaudry JS. Effectiveness of continuing Medical Education: a quantitative synthesis. *J Contin Educ Health.* 1989; **9**: 285–307.

Becher T. The Learning Professions. *Stud High Educ.* 1996; **21**(1): 43–55.

Bell G. *A study which explores the feasibility of establishing general practice as multi-disciplinary training practices.* Unpublished report. Sunderland Health Authority; 1996.

Bellack JP. Characteristics and outcomes of a statewide nurse refresher project. *J Contin Educ Nurs.* 1995; **26**(2): 60–6.

Benett, Y. The validity and reliability of assessment and self-assessments of work-based learning. *Assessment and Evaluation in Higher Education.* 1993; **18**: 83–94.

Bennett NL, Casebeer LL. Evolution of planning in CME. *J Contin Educ Health.* 1995; **15**: 70–9.

Bertram DA, Brooks-Bertram PA. The evaluation of continuing Medical Education: a literature review. *Health Educ Mono.* 1997; **5**: 330–62.

Biddle C. AANA journal course: update for nurse anesthetists – outcome measures in anesthesiology: are we going in the right direction? *AANA J.* 1994; **62**(2): 117–24.

Blanchard D, Fox RD. A Profile of nonurban physicians from the study of changing and learning in the lives of physicians. *J Contin Educ Health.* 1990; **10**: 329–38.

Bloom BS. Effects of continuing Medical Education on improving physician clinical care and patient health: a review of systematic reviews. *Int J Technol Assess.* 2005; **21**(3): 380–5.

Boud DC. How to Help Students Learn from Experience. In: Al-Shehri, *et al.*, 1993 op.cit.

BPMF. *The Quality of Continuing Med Educ for General Practitioners.* London: British Post-graduate Medical Federation; 1993.

Brady L. Assessing curriculum outcomes in Australian schools. *Educ Rev.* 1997; **49**: 57–65.

Branthwaite A, Ross A, Henshaw A, *et al.* Continuing Education for General Practitioners. *Occasional Paper 38.* London; Royal College of General Practitioners; 1988.

Brookfield SD. *Understanding and Facilitating Adult Learning.* Buckingham: Open University Press; 1986.

Burge EJ, and others. The Audioconference: Delivering continuing education for addictions workers in Canada. *J Alcohol Drug Educ.* 1993; **39**(1): 78–91.

Burrows P. Continuing Medical Education and pharmaceutical sponsorship. *Postgrad Educ Gen Pract.* 1990; **1**: 115–16.

Byers DL, and others. Evaluation of interactive television continuing education programs for health-care professionals. *J Educ Technol Systems.* 1996; **24**(3): 259–70.

Campbell C, Gondocz T, Parboosingh IJT. Documenting and managing self-directed learning among specialists. *Ann Roy Coll Physic.* 1995; **28**: 80–4.

Cantwell ZM. School-based leadership and professional socialization of the assistant principal. *Urban Education.* 1993; **28**(1): 49–68.

Carr A. Clinical psychology in Ireland – a national survey. *Irish J Psychol.* 1995; **16**(1): 1–20.

Cervero RM. *Effective Continuing Education for Professionals.* San Francisco: Jossey-Bass; 1988.

Cervero RM. The importance of practical knowledge and implications for continuing education. *J Contin Educ Health.* 1990; **10**: 85–94.

Cervero RM, Rottet S. Analyzing the effectiveness of continuing professional education: an exploratory study. *Adult Educ Quart.* 1984; **34**: 135–46.

Challis M, Mathers NJ, Howe AC, *et al.* Portfolio-based learning: continuing Medical Education for general practitioners – a mid-point evaluation. *Med Educ.* 1997; 31, 22–6.

Chambers E. *Mentoring, Self-directed Learning, and Continuing Professional Education.* Milton Keynes: The Open University; 1992.

Charlton G. Megatrials are based on a methodological mistake. *Brit J Gen Pract.* 1996; **46**: 429–31.

Cividin TM, Ottoson JM. Linking reasons for continuing professional education participation with postprogram application. *J Contin Educ Health.* 1997; **17**: 46–55.

Conway AC, Keller RB, Wennberg DE. Partnering with physicians to achieve quality improvement. *Joint Comm J Qual Im.* 1995; **21**(11): 619–26.

Cornell JM, Kahn EH, Bahrawy AA. The school nurse development program: An experiment in off-site delivery. *J Contin Educ Nurs.* 1992; **23**(3): 127–33.

Crandall SJS. The role of continuing Medical Education in changing and learning. *J Contin Educ Health.* 1990; **10**: 339–48.

Crandall SJS, Cunliff AE. Experience with mandatory continuing education in a teaching hospital. *J Contin Educ Health.* 1989; 9: 155–63.

Curran V, Rourke L, Snow P. A framework for enhancing continuing Medical Education for rural physicians:a summary of the literature. *Med Teach.* 2010; **32**: e501 – e508. (web paper)

D'Alessandro MP, Galvin JR, Erkonen WE, *et al.* The virtual hospital: an IAIMS continuing education into the work flow. *MD Computing.* 1996; **13**(4): 323–29.

Dall'Alba G, Sandberg J. Educating for Competence in Professional Practice. *Instr Sci.* 1996; **24**: 411–37.

Dalton JA, Blau W, Carlson J, *et al.* Changing the relationship among nurses' knowledge, self-reported behavior, and documented behavior in pain management: does education make a difference? *J Pain Symptom Manag.* 1996; **12**(5): 308–19.

Davidson R, Sensakovic J, Helm C, *et al.* The Effect of CME on Physicians' Counseling, Testing, and Management of HIV Infection. *J Contin Educ Health.* 1990; **10**: 303–13.

Davis DA. A Critical Analysis of the Literature Evaluating CME. *Möbius.* 1987; **7**: 87–95.

Davis D. Does CME work? An analysis of the effect of educational activities on physician performance or health care outcomes. *Int J Psychiat Med.* 1998; **28**(1): 21–39.

Davis D, Thomson MA. Implications for undergraduate and graduate education derived from quantitative research in continuing Medical Education: lessons learned from an automobile. *J Contin Educ Health.* 1996; **16**: 159–66.

Davis DA, Thomson MA, Oxman AD, *et al.* Changing physician performance: a systematic review of the effect of continuing Medical Education strategies. *JAMA.* 1995; **274**: 700–5.

Davis DA, Thomson MA, Oxmon AD, *et al.* Evidence for the effectiveness of CME: a review of 50 randomized control trials. *JAMA.* 1992; **268**: 1111–17.

Davis MH, Harden RM, Laidlaw JM, *et al.* Continuing education for general dental practitioners using a printed distance learning programme. *Med Educ.* 1992; **26**: 378–83.

De Buda Y, Woolf CR. Saturday at the university: A format for success. *J Contin Educ Health.* 1990; **10**: 279–84.

DoH. *The National Health Service: A Service with Ambitions.* London: HMSO; 1996a.

DoH. *Primary Care: Choice and Opportunity.* London: HMSO; 1996b.

DoH. *Primary Care: Delivering the Future.* London: HMSO; 1996c.

DoH. *Learning from Bristol; The Report of the Public Inquiry into Children's Heart Surgery at the Bristol Royal Infirmary, 1984–1995,* CM5207; 2001.

DoH and the Welsh Office. *General Practice in the National Health Service: A new contract.* London: HMSO; 1989.

Docking S. Professional development through distance learning: the professional nurses accredited learning scheme. *Prof Nurs.* 1993; **9**(1): 38–41.

DoH. *Consultation Paper for the Chief Medical Officer's Conference on Continuing Education for Doctors and Dentists.* Working Document. Department of Health; 1995.

Dunn WR, Hamilton DD. Competence-based education and distance learning: a tandem for professional continuing education. *Stud High Educ.* 1985; **10**: 277–87.

Durno D, Gill GM. Survey of general practitioners' views on postgraduate education in North-East Scotland. *J R Coll Gen Pract.* 1974; **24**: 648–54.

Ebel R. The practical validation of tests of ability. *Educational Measurement: Issues and Practice,* 1983; **2**: 7–10.

Emens JM. *Intractible Vaginal Discharge.* PACE Review for the Royal College of Obstetricians and Gynaecologists; 1995.

Eraut, M. Do continuing professional models promote one-dimensional learning? *Med Educ.* 2001; **35**: 8–11.

Falvo DR. Educational evaluation: what are the outcomes? *Adv Renal Replac Th.* 1995; 2(3): 227–33.

Feder GS, Griffiths, CJ, Grimshaw JM. (1997). Healthcare practice guidelines for chronic disease management. Do they change practice? *Dis Manag Health Out.* 1997; **1**(3): 129–34.

Feest T. NVQs in publishing – why bother? *Learn Publ.* 1996; **9**(2): 79–85.

Ferguson A. Evaluating the purpose and benefits of continuing education in nursing and the implications for the provision of continuing education for cancer nurses. *J Adv Nurs.* 1994; **19**(4): 640–6.

Fish D, Coles C. *Learning through the Critical Appreciation of Practice.* Butterworth Heinemann, London; 1998.

Fleming RM, Fleming DM, Gaede R. Training physicians and health care providers to accurately read coronary arteriograms. A training program. *Angiology.* 1996; **47**(4): 349–59.

Fox RD. New horizons for research in continuing Medical Education. *Acad Med.* 1990; **65**(9): 550–5.

Fox RD, Mazmanian PE, Putnam WR. *Changing and Learning in the Lives of Physicians.* New York: Praeger; 1989.

Francis BW, Fisher CC. Multilevel library instruction for emerging nursing roles. *B Med Libr Assoc.* 1995; **83**(4): 492–8.

Gale R, Grant J. AMEE Medical Education guide. No.10: managing change in a medical context. Guidelines for action. *Med Teach.* 1997; **19**(4): 239–49.

Gear J, McIntosh A, Squires G. *Informal Learning in the Professions.* Hull: University of Hull; 1994.

General Medical Council. *Guidance on CPD*; 2001. www.gmc-uk.org/education/continuing_professional_development/cpd_guidance.asp

Gerrard J, Holden JM, Elliott SA. A trainer's perspective of an innovative program teaching health visitors about the detection, treatment and prevention of postnatal depression. *J Adv Nurs.* 1993; **18**(11): 1825–32.

Hammick M, Freeth D, Koppel I, *et al.* A best evidence systematic review of interprofessional education BEME guide no. 9. *Med Teach.* 2008; **29**(8): 735–51.

Gibbs G, Morgan A, Taylor E. *The World of the Learner.* In: Al-Shehri, *et al.,* 1993. op. cit.

Glazier R, Buchbinder R, Bell M. Critical appraisal of continuing Medical Education in the rheumatic diseases for primary care physicians. *Arthritis Rheumatol.* 1995; **38**(4): 533–8.

Glazier RH, Dalby DM, Badley EM, *et al.* Determinants of physician confidence in the primary care management of musculoskeletal disorders. *J Rheumatol.* 1996; **23**(2): 351–6.

Goodsman D. *Continuing Professional Development*. London: Joint Centre for Education in Medicine; 1994.

Gottfried SS, Kyle WC. Textbook use and the biology education desired state. *J Res Sci Teach*. 1992; **29**(1): 35–49.

Graham I. I believe therefore I practise. *Lancet*. 1996; **347**: 4–5.

Grant J. CME: Its validation and outcome. In: Mansfield; 1994. op.cit.

Grant J, Stanton F, Flood S, *et al. An Evaluation of Educational Needs and Provision for Doctors within Three Years of Completion of Training*. Joint Centre for Education in Medicine, London; 1998.

Gray DP. Continuing education for general practitioners. *J R Coll Gen Pract*. 1988; May, 195–6.

Green LW, Kreuter MW. *Health Promotion Planning: An educational and environmental approach*. Mountain View; California: Mayfield; 1991.

Green L, Kreuter M, Deeds S, *et al. Health Education Planning: A diagnostic approach*. Palo Alto; California: Mayfield Press; 1980.

Grilli R, Lomas J. Evaluating the message: the relationship between compliance rate and subject of a practice guideline. *Med Care*. 1994; **32**: 202–13.

Gross SM. Demographic study of the relationship of continuing pharmaceutical education to selected attitudinal- and competence-related criteria. *Am J Pharm Educ*. 1976; **40**: 141–8.

Grotelveschen AD, Hamish DL, Kenny WR. *An analysis of the participation reasons scale administered to business professionals*. occasional paper 7. Urbana: Office for the Study of Continuing Professional Education, University of Illinois at Urbana-Champaign; 1979.

Hadiyono JE, Suryawati S, Danu SS, *et al*. Interactional group discussion: results of a controlled trial using a behavioral intervention to reduce the use of injections in public health facilities. *Soc Sci Med*. 1996; **42**(8): 1177–83.

Hager P, Gonczi A, Athanasou J. General issues about assessment of competence. *Assessment and Evaluation in Higher Education*. 1994; **19**: 3–16.

Harden RM, Laidlaw JM. Effective continuing education: The CRISIS criteria. *Med Educ*. 1992; **26**: 408–22.

Harmes HM, Sullivan DE. A study of long-term outcomes of return-to-industry programs. *Community Coll Rev*. 1994; **22**(2): 48–54.

Harrison, B. CME: A trust view. In: Mansfield, op.cit.

Havener WM, Worrell P. Environmental factors in professional development activities – Does type of academic library affiliation make a difference? *Libr Inform Sci Res*. 1994; **16**(3): 318–20.

Headrick L, Katcher W, Neuhauser D, *et al*. Continuous quality improvement and knowledge for improvement applied to asthma care. *Joint Comm J Qual Im*. 1994; **20**(10): 562–8.

Hedman L, Lazure LA. Extending continuing education to rural area nurses. *J Contin Educ Nurs*. 1990; **21**(4): 165–8.

Helsby G. Defining and developing professionalism in English secondary schools. *J Educ Teaching*. 1996; **22**(2): 135–8.

Hoftvedt BO, Mjell J. Referrals: Peer review as continuing Medical Education. *Teach Learn Med*. 1993; **5**(4): 234–7.

Hoftvedt BO, Paus A, Natrud E, *et al*. Evaluating a management training program for hospital doctors in Norway. *J Contin Educ Health*. 1995; **15**: 91–4.

Hollwitz J, Danielson MA. Measure the place before you measure the people: new alternatives for quality assessment. *Assessment and Evaluation in Higher Education.* 1995; **20:** 67–76.

Houle CO. *Continuing Learning in the Professions.* San Francisco: Jossey-Bass; 1980.

Hughes RB, Cummings H, Allen RV. The nurse *extern practicum*: a new partnership between education and service. *JNSD.* 1993; 9(3): 118–21.

Iphofen R, Poland F. Professional empowerment and Teach Sociology to health care professionals. *Teach Sociol.* 1997; **25**(1): 44–56.

Jackson BJ, Hays BJ, Robinson CC. Multiple delivery methods for an interdisciplinary audience: assessing effectiveness. *J Contin Educ Health.* 1990; **10:** 59–69.

Jacobsen C, Malan S, Perkins T, *et al.* A regional approach to entry-level critical care education. *Focus Critical Care.* 1990; **17**(5): 385–6.

Jacobson LD, Edwards AE, Granier SK, *et al.* Evidence-based medicine and general practice. *Brit J Gen Pract.* 1997; **47:** 449–52.

Jansen JJM, Tan LHC, van der Vleuten CPM, *et al.* Assessment of competence in technical clinical skills of general practitioners. *Med Educ.* 1995; **25:** 414–20.

Jansen JJM, Scherpbier AJJA, Metz JCM, *et al.* Performance-based assessment in continuing Medical Education for general practitioners: construct validity. *Med Educ.* 1996; **30:** 339–44.

Järvinin A, Konoven V. Promoting professional development in higher education through portfolio assessment. *Assessment and Evaluation in Higher Education.* 1995; **20:** 25–36.

Jasper MA. The potential of the professional portfolio for nursing. *J Clin Nurs.* 1995; 4(4): 249–55.

Jennett PA, Scott SM, Atkinson MA, *et al.* Patients charts and physician office management decisions: chart audit and chart stimulated recall. *J Contin Educ Health.* 1995; **15:** 31–9.

Jennett PA, Laxdal OE, Hayton RC, *et al.* The effects of continuing Medical Education on family doctor performance in office practice: a randomised control study. *Med Educ.* 1988; **22:** 139–45.

Johns C, Graham J. The growth of management connoisseurship through reflective practice. *J Nurs Man.* 1994; 2(6): 253–60.

Joint Centre for Education in Medicine. *Assessing and improving in general practice. Feasibility study.* Confidential report to the NHSE Development Unit; 1997.

Jolly B, Grant J. *Good Assessment Guide.* London: Joint Centre for Education in Medicine; 1997. oucem@open.ac.uk

Jones N, Fear N. Continuing professional development – Perspectives from human-resource professionals. *Pers Rev.* 1994; **23**(8): 49–60.

Kalnins I, Phelps SL, Glauber W. Outcomes of nurse (RN) refresher courses in a midwestern city. *J Contin Educ Nurs.* 1994; **25**(6): 268–271.

Kelly MH, Murray TS. Who are the providers of Medical Education? *Med Educ.* 1993; **27:** 452–60.

Kelly MH, Murray TS. Motivation of general practitioners attending postgraduate education. *Brit J Gen Pract.* 1996; **46:** 353–6.

Kerr DNS. *The Value of CME.* Abstracts of the Second Conference held at the Royal Society in Medicine: 'British Continuing Medical Education: A framework for the future' (15th and 16th Sep); 1994.

Klayman J, Brown K. Debias the environment instead of the judge: An alternative approach to reducing error in diagnostic (and other) judgment. *Cognition.* 1993; **49**(1–2): 97–122.

Knowles MS. *Self-directed Learning: A guide for learners and teachers.* New York: Cambridge Books; 1975.

Knox AB. Influences on participation in continuing education. *J Contin Educ Health.*1990; **19**(3): 261–74.

Kopp ME, Schell KA, Laskowski-Jones L, *et al.* Crit Care Nurse internships: in theory and practice. *Crit Care Nurse.* 1993; **13**(4): 115–18.

Kuramoto, AM, Wyman JA. Design and implementation of effective delivery approaches for continuing nursing education. *Möbius.* 1986; **6**: 6–10.

Kushnir T, Vigiser D, Weisberg, E, *et al.* A graduate course in work site health promotion for occupational health practitioners. *Journal Occup Environ Med.* 1996; **38**(3): 284–9.

Lane DS. Outcome measurement in multi-interventional continuing Medical Education. *J Contin Educ Health.* 1997; **17**: 12–19.

Langham S, Gillam S, Thorogood M. 'The carrot, the stick, and the general practitioner: how have changes in financial incentives affected health promotion in general practice?' *Brit J Gen Pract.* 1995; **45**: 665–8.

Langsner SJ. Deterrents to participation in continuing professional education: a survey of the NTRS. *Therap Rec J.* 1994; **28**(3): 147–62.

Laxdal OE. Needs assessment in continuing Medical Education: a practical guide. *J Med Educ.* 1982; **57**: 827–34.

Lewis AP, Bolden KJ. General practitioners and their learning styles. *J R Coll Gen Pract.* 1989; **39**: 187–9.

Lexchin J. Interactions between physicians and the pharmaceutical industry: what does the literature say? *Can Med Assoc J.* 1993; **149**(10): 1401–7.

Loughridge B, Oates J, Speight S. Career Development – Follow-up studies of Sheffield MA graduates 1985/1986 to 1992/1993. *J Libr Inf Sci.* 1996; **28**(2): 105–17.

Madlon-Kay DJ. Improvement in family physician recognition and treatment of hypercholesterolemia. *Arch Intern Med.* 1989; **149**: 1754–5.

Malenka DJ, O'Connor GT. A regional collaborative effort for CQI in cardiovascular disease. Northern New England cardiovascular study group. *Joint Comm J Qual Im.* 1995; **21**(11): 627–33.

Mann KV, Langille DB, Weld VP, *et al.* Multidisciplinary learning in continuing professional education: the heart health Nova Scotia experience. *J Contin Educ Health.* 1996; **16**: 50–60.

Mansfield A. *CME and the Royal College of Surgeons.* Abstracts of the 1st conference held at the Royal Society of Medicine: 'British Continuing Medical Education: A framework for the future.' (4th and 5th Jul); 1994.

Mayne K. Practice-linked continuing Medical Education. *Med J Australia.* 1994; **161**(10): 630–2.

Mazmanian PE, Williams RB, Desch CE. Theory and research for the development of continuing education in the health professions. *J Contin Educ Health.* 1990; **10**: 349–65.

Mazmanian PE. Continuing Medical Education and the physician as a learner. *JAMA.* 2002; 4th Sep, **288**(9): 1057–60.

McAuley RG, Paul WM, Morrison GH, *et al.* Five-Year results of the peer assessment program of the college of physicians and surgeons of Ontario. *Can Med Assoc J.* 1990; **143**: 1193–9.

McClennan BL, Herlihy CS. The continuing competence needs of physicians: a survey of the medical specialty societies. *Am J Roentgenol.* 1995; **165**(4): 789–96.

McGuire C. The Curriculum for the Year 2000. *Med Educ.* 1989; **23**: 221–7.

McKinley WJD. (1990). *Continuing Medical Education 19th century style: the role of the New Sydenham Society in the education of doctors in North West England in 1866.* Proceedings of the XXXIInd International Congress on the History of Medicine, Antwerp.

McKnight A, Bradley T. How do general practitioners qualify for their PGEA? *Brit J Gen Pract.* 1996; **46**: 679–80.

Melton R. Learning outcomes for higher education: some key issues. *Brit J Educ Stud.* 1996; **44**: 409–25.

Millar C. Educating the educators of adults: Two cheers for curriculum negotiation. *J Curriculum Stud.* 1989; **21**: 161–8.

Moore DE. Moving CME close to the clinical encounter: the promise of quality management and CME. *J Contin Educ Health.* 1995; **15**: 135–45.

Moore P, Pace KB, Rapacz K. Collaborative model for continuing education for home health nurses. *J Contin Educ Nurs.* 1991; **22**(2): 67–72.

Morrow NC, Hargie ODW. Influencing and persuading skills at the interprofessional interface: training for action. *J Contin Educ Health.* 1996; **16**: 94–102.

Murdock JE, Neafsey PJ. Self-Efficacy Measurements: an approach for predicting practice outcomes in continuing education? *J Contin Educ Nurs.* 1995; **26**(4): 158–65.

Murray TS, Dyker GS, Campbell LM. Characteristics of general practitioners who are high attenders at educational meetings. *Brit J Gen Pract.* 1992; **42**: 157–9.

Murray TS, Dyker GS, Campbell LM. Continuing Medical Education and the education allowance: variation in credits obtained by GPs. *Med Educ.* 1992; **26**: 248–50.

Murray TS, Dyker GS, Campbell LM. Postgraduate education allowance: general practitioners' attendance at courses outwith their region. *Brit J Gen Pract.* 1992; **42**: 194–6.

NHS Scotland *Making Continuing Professional Development Work*; 2003.

Norman GR, van der Vleuten CPM, de Graaf E. Pitfalls in the pursuit of objectivity: issues of validity, efficiency and acceptability. *Med Educ.* 1991; **25**: 119–26.

Nowlem PM. *A New Approach to Continuing Education for Business and the Professions.* New York: MacMillan; 1988.

Okey A, Wood F, Lawes A. Surveying the effectiveness of short-course provision in the professional development of library and information specialists. *J Educ Libr Inf Sci.* 1992; **33**(3): 249–53.

Ottoson JM. Use of a conceptual framework to explore multiple influences on the application of learning following a continuing education program. *Can J Study Adult Learning.* 1995; **9**: 1–18.

Paget NS, Saunders NA, Newble NA, *et al.* Physician assessment pilot study for the Royal Australasian College of Physicians. *J Contin Educ Health.* 1996; **16**: 103–11.

Parboosingh IJT. Learning portfolios: potential to assist health professionals with self-directed learning. *J Contin Educ Health.* 1996; **16**: 75–81.

Parboosingh IJT, Campbell CM, Gondocz T. Development of a standard for self-directed continuing Medical Education. *Ann Roy Coll Physic.* 1995; **28**: 75–8.

Parboosingh IJT, Gondocz ST, Lai A. The annual MOCOMP profile. *Ann Roy Coll Physic.* 1993; **26**: 544–7.

Parboosingh IJT, Thivierge RL. The Maintenance of Competence (MOCOMP) Program. *Ann Roy Coll Physic.* 1993; **26**: 512–17.

Parker DJ, Gray HH, Balcon R, *et al.* Planning for Coronary Angioplasty: Guidelines for training and continuing competence. British Cardiac Society (BCS) and British Cardiovascular Intervention Society (BCIS) working group on interventional cardiology. *Heart.* 1996; **75**(4): 419–25.

Pearson P, Jones K. Developing professional knowledge: making primary course education and research more relevant. *BMJ.* 1997; **314**: 817–20.

Pickup AJ, Mee LG, Hedley AJ. The general practitioner and continuing education. *Brit J Gen Pract.* 1983; **33**: 486–92.

Pinion SB. *Conservative Alternatives to Hysterectomy for Dysfunctional Uterine Bleeding.* PACE Review for the Royal College of Obstetricians and Gynaecologists; 1994.

Piterman L. GPs as learners. *Med J Australia.* 1991; **155**: 318–22.

Pories WJ, Smout JC, Morris A, *et al.* U.S. health care reform: will it change postgraduate surgical education? *World J Surg.* 1994; **18**(5): 745–52.

Purnell L. Outcomes of a university-based registered nurse refresher course: a 5-year follow-up. *JNSD.* 1995; **11**(1): 31–4.

RACGP. *Quality Assurance and Continuing Education Programme 1993–1995.* Rozelle; NSW: Royal Australian College of General Practitioners; 2001.

Ramsden P. *Improving Learning: New perspectives.* London: Kogan Page; 1988.

Raymond M. *Continuing Education in the Health Professions: A reanalysis of the literature.* Paper presented at the meeting of the American Educational Research Association, San Francisco; 1986.

RCOGS. *CME Credit Book.* London: Royal College of Obstetricians and Gynaecologists; 1994.

RCP. *Continuing Medical Education for the Trained Physician: Recommendations for the introduction and implementation of a CME system.* The Royal Colleges of Physicians of Edinburgh, Glasgow and London; 1994.

Reedy BLEC. General practitioners and postgraduate education in the Northern Region: occasional paper 9. 1979; *J R Coll Gen Pract.*

Robb AJP, Murray R. Medical humanities in nursing – thought provoking. *J Adv Nurs.* 1992; **17**(10): 1182–7.

Rogers A. Learning: can we change the discourse? *Adults Learning.* 1997; Jan, 116–17.

Rogers EM. *Diffusion of Innovations.* New York: Free Press; 1983.

Rolfe IE, Andrei JM, Pearson S, *et al.* Clinical competence of interns. *Med Educ.* 1995; **29**: 225–30.

Royal College of General Practitioners. Occasional paper 50. *Fellowship by Assessment.* 2nd ed. Exeter: RCGP; 1995.

Royal College of Nursing *Quality Education for Quality Care. Priorities and Actions;* 2002. www.rcn.org.uk/data/assets/pdf_file/0006/78612/002297.pdf

RSM. *Yearbook of Continuing Medical Education 1995.* London: The Royal Society of Medicine Press; 1995.

Sandars J. Cost-effective continuing professional development. In: K Walsh (ed.). *Cost Effectiveness in Medical Education.* Oxford: Radcliffe Publishing; 2010.

Sandmire HF, DeMott RK. The Green Bay Cesarean Section Study.III. Falling cesarean birth rates without a formal curtailment program. *Am J Obstet Gynecol.* 1994; **170**(6): 1790–9.

Saul JL. Action outcome evaluation: a case study. *J Contin Higher Educ.* 1992; **40**(1): 18–21.

Saywell RM, Jay SJ, Lukas PJ, *et al.* Indiana family physician attitudes and practices concerning smoking cessation. *Indiana Med.* 1996; **89**(2): 149–56.

Scheller MK. A qualitative analysis of factors in the work environment that influence nurses' use of knowledge gained from CE programs. *J Contin Educ Nurs.* 1993; **24**(3): 114–22.

Schön D. *Educating the Reflective Practitioner* (2nd ed.). San Francisco: Jossey-Bass; 1987.

Schostak J, Davis M, Hanson J, *et al. The Effectiveness of Continuing Professional Development. Final Report.* Academy of Medical Royal Colleges and General Medical Council. London; 2010. www.aomrc.org.uk/publications/reports-guidance.html

SCMCDCME. *Future Directions for Medical College Continuing Medical Education.* Washington: Society of Medical Directors of CME; 1995.

Seitz JA. A collaborative approach to professional development. *J Contin Higher Educ.* 1995; **43**(1): 44–53.

Shenk D, Lee J. Meeting the educational needs of service providers: effects of a continuing education program on self-reported knowledge and attitudes about aging. *Educ Gerontol,* 1995; **21**(7): 671–81.

Shirriffs G. Continuing educational requirements for general practitioners in Grampian. *J R Coll Gen Pract.* 1989; **39**: 190–2.

Sibley JC, Sackett DL, Neufeld V, *et al.* A randomized control trial of continuing Medical Education. *New Engl J Med.* 1982; **306**: 511–15.

Singleton A, Tylee A. Continuing Medical Education in mental illness: a paradox for general practitioners. *Brit J Gen Pract.* 1996; **46**: 339–41.

SMA. *Continuing Medical Education in Sweden: An education policy programme.* Stockholm: Swedish Medical Association; 1995.

Stanley I, Al-Shehri A, Thomas P. Continuing education for general practice. 1. Experience, competence and the media of self-directed learning for established general practitioners. *Brit J Gen Pract.* 1993; **43**: 210–14.

Stanton F, Grant J. *Approaches to Experiential Learning in Medicine. A Background Document.* Joint Centre for Education in Medicine, London. ISBN 1873207 91 3; 1998.

Stokes RA. Streamlining orientation for haemodialysis nursing: a competency-based approach. *ANNA J.* 1991; **18**(1): 33–8.

Stross GK. Relationships between knowledge and experience in the use of disease-modifying antirheumatic agents: a study of primary care practitioners. *JAMA.* 1989; **19**: 2721–3.

Sullivan F, Mitchell E. Has general practitioner computing made a difference to patient care? A systematic review of published reports. *BMJ.* 1995; **311**: 848–52.

The Mackinnon Partnership.*A Literature Review of the Relationship between Quality Health Care Education and Quality of Care. A report to Skills for Health;* 2007. www.themackinnonpartnership.co.uk

Tjeltveit AC. The psychotherapist as Christian ethicist – theology applied to practice. *J Psychol Theol.* 1992; **20**(2): 89–98.

Todd F. (Ed.). *Planning Continuing Professional Development.* London: Croom Helm; 1987.

Tolnai S. Continuing Medical Education and career choice among graduates of problem-based and traditional curricula. *Med Educ.* 1991; **25**: 414–20.

Tracey JM, Arroll B, Richmond DE, *et al.* The validity of general practitioners' self-assessment of knowledge: cross sectional study. *BMJ.* 1997; **315**: 1426–8.

Tulinius C, Holge-Hazelton B. Continuing professional development for general practitioners: supporting the development of professionalism. *Med Educ.* 2010; **44**: 412–20.

Tunstall-Pedoe S, Rink E, Hilton S. Student attitudes to undergraduate interprofessional education. *J Interprofessional Care.* 2003; **17**(2): 161–72.

UEMS. *Charter on Continuing Medical Education of Medical Specialists in the European Union.* Brussels: Union Européenne des Médicins Specialistes; 1994.

UEMS. *Basel Declaration. UEMS Policy on Continuing Professional Development;* 2001. http://admin.uems.net/uploadedfiles/35.pdf

UEMS.*The Accreditation of e-Learning Materials by the EACCME;* 2008. http://admin.uems.net/uploadedfiles/1177.pdf

van der Vleuten CPM. The assessment of professional competence: developments, research and practical implications. *Adv Health Sci Educ.* 1996; **1**: 41–67.

van der Vleuten CPM, Norman GR, de Graaf E. Pitfalls in the pursuit of objectivity: issues of reliability. *Med Educ.* 1991; **25**: 110–18.

Van Harrison R, Gallay LS, McKay NE, *et al.* The association between community physicians' attendance at a medical centre's CME courses and their patient referrals to the medical centre. *J Contin Educ Health.* 1990; **10**: 315–20.

Vaughan P. *Maintaining Professional Competence: A survey of the role of professional bodies in the development of credit-bearing CPD courses.* Hull: University of Hull; 1991.

Vickrey BG. Outcomes research – possible effects on clinical practice. *Western J Med.* 1993; **159**(2): 183–4.

Volberding PA. Improving the outcomes of care for patients with human immunodeficiency virus infection. *New Engl J Med.* 1996; **334**(11): 729–31.

Walsh JME, McPhee SJ. A systems model for clinical preventive care: an analysis of factors influencing patient and physician. *Health Educ Quart.* 1992; **19**: 157–75.

Walton HJ. Continuing Medical Education and changes in doctors. *Med Educ.* 1991; **25**: 1–2.

Walton HJ. Continuing Medical Education in Europe: a survey. *Med Educ.* 1994; **28**: 333–42.

Weerakoon PK, Fernando DN. Self-evaluation of skills as a method of assessing learning needs for continuing education. *Med Teach.* 1991; **13**: 103–6.

Wergin JF, Mazmanian PE, Miller WW, *et al.* CME and change in practice: an alternative perspective. *J Contin Educ Health.* 1988; **8**: 147–59.

Wilbur RS. Report: 1st International Conference on Continuing Medical Education. Rancho Mirage, California, 30 November–4 December 1986. *Med Educ.* 1987; **21**(2): 157–64.

Wiles R. Quality questions. *Nurs Times.* 1996; October 30, **92**(44): 38–40.

Williams AR, Davis RD, Hale CD, *et al.* Patterns of concern: needs assessment and continuing education needs among public health physicians. *J Contin Educ Health.* 1989; **9**: 131–9.

Williamson JW, German PS, Weiss R, *et al.* Health science information management and continuing education of physicians: a survey of US primary care practitioners and their opinion leaders. *Ann Intern Med.* 1989; **110**: 151–60.

Wood J, Byrne PS. Section 63 activities: occasional paper 11. *J R Coll Gen Pract.* 1980.

Woolf CR. Personal continuing education relationships between perceived needs by individual physicians and practice profiles. *J Contin Educ Health.* 1988; **8**: 271–6.

Woolf CR. Personal Continuing Education (PECE) plan: stage 2 – a model to supply physicians' perceived needs. *J Contin Educ Health.* 1990; **10**: 321–8.

Young Y, Brigley S, Littlejohns P, *et al.* Continuing education for public health medicine – is it just another paper exercise? *J Public Health Med.* 1996; **18**(3): 357–63.

Appendix 2: Appraisal record form template

THE APPRAISAL PROCESS

During the appraisal, the appraiser and doctor might keep a note of the conclusions of each section. An example of an Appraisal Record Form, for use by the doctor and/or appraiser is given on the next page. This should be completed during the appraisal meeting. The order of the appraisal meeting or professional conversation might be as follows:

Topic	Person being appraised	Appraiser/peer
Overview	How does the doctor view his/her work since the last meeting? Was the previous CPD plan achieved?	How does the appraiser view the doctor's work since the last meeting?
Description	How would the doctor describe his/her performance in the last year?	How would the appraiser describe the doctor's performance in the last year?
Positive evaluation	What did the doctor do well? How does he/she know?	What did the doctor do well? How does the appraiser know?
Personal learning needs	What personal learning needs does the doctor now have? How does the doctor know? *The doctor might have identified a personal learning need by any of the means described in Part Three below or in other ways.*	What did not go so well? How does the appraiser know?
Service needs	Is there any other CPD the doctor would like to undertake in relation to plans for service development?	Is there any other CPD the doctor should undertake in relation to plans for service development?

continued

Topic	Person being appraised	Appraiser/peer
CPD activities	What CPD would the doctor like to undertake now? *The doctor might elect to undertake CPD in any of the ways described in Step Three or in other ways.*	
Reinforcement/ dissemination follow-up plans	How does the doctor plan to locally reinforce and disseminate the CPD once it is completed? *The doctor might choose any of the ways described in Step Four or in other ways.*	
Practical planning	How and when will the CPD be organised? When will the study leave application be made?	

APPRAISAL RECORD FORM

Doctor:	
Appraiser/peer:	
Date:	

Topic	Record of conversation/decisions
Overview of the year, including achievement of previous plan	
Description of performance	
Positive evaluation: What went well	

continued

Topic	Record of conversation/decisions
Personal learning needs/wants identified	
Service needs identified	
CPD activities planned	
Reinforcement/dissemination/follow-up plans made	
Practical planning: organisation of CPD activities/study leave application	

Appendix 3: Methods of needs assessment

Clinicians use many ways of assessing their own educational needs. The following methods of assessing a clinician's CPD needs are described and evaluated in Step One.

TYPE	*METHOD*
The clinician's own experiences in direct patient care	➤ Blind spots ➤ Clinically-generated unknowns ➤ Competence standards ➤ Diaries ➤ Difficulties arising in practice ➤ Innovations in practice ➤ Knowledgeable patients ➤ Mistakes ➤ Other disciplines ➤ Patients' complaints and feedback ➤ Post-mortems and the clinico-pathological conference (CPC) ➤ PUNs and DENs ➤ Reflection on practical experience
Interactions within the clinical team and department	➤ Clinical meetings: departmental and grand rounds ➤ Department business plan ➤ Department educational meetings ➤ External recruitment ➤ Junior staff ➤ Management roles ➤ Mentoring
Non-clinical activities	➤ Academic activities ➤ Conferences ➤ International visits ➤ Journal articles ➤ Medico-legal cases ➤ Press and media ➤ Professional conversations ➤ Research ➤ Teaching

continued

TYPE	*METHOD*
Formal approaches to quality management and risk assessment	➤ Audit ➤ Morbidity patterns ➤ Patient adverse events ➤ Patient satisfaction surveys ➤ Risk assessment ➤ Portfolios
Specific activities directed at needs assessment	➤ Critical incident surveys ➤ Gap analysis ➤ Objective tests of knowledge and skill ➤ Observation ➤ Revalidation systems ➤ Self-assessment ➤ Video assessment of performance
Peer review	➤ External peer review ➤ Informal peer review of the individual doctor ➤ Internal peer review ➤ Multidisciplinary peer review ➤ Physician assessment (360 degree assessment, multisource feedback)

Appendix 4: A study leave application form

Name:		Department:	
Date of appraisal:		Name of appraiser:	
DATES OF PROPOSED STUDY LEAVE:		From:	
		To:	

	Local (specify):
Location of study:	Non-local (specify):
	Abroad (specify):

Nature of study leave activity:	
Relevance of this activity to your work/department:	Personal relevance:
	Service relevance:

How will you follow-up the study leave?	
Is the proposed activity approved …	By your professional body? (specify):
	With an appraiser or peer? (specify):

Does the activity fit into a defined CPD category?	Specify:
If yes, how many points/credits/hours have you applied for?	

Is cover required for your work duties?	Yes No

IF YES:	
Who is providing cover?	
How many clinics cancelled?	
How many ward rounds cancelled?	
How many lists cancelled?	
How many other types of session cancelled? (specify type)	

ESTIMATED COSTS OF STUDY LEAVE:	
Registration fee:	
Accommodation:	
Travel:	
Subsistence:	
Other (specify):	
Total:	
What other sources of financial support are available?	

SIGNATURE:..........................

Date:..................................

Administrative approval:	*Professional approval:*
Signature:	*Signature:*
Date:	*Date:*

Please submit this to the relevant person for processing. Lodge a copy in your portfolio.

Appendix 5: Methods of professional learning

Clinicians have many ways of learning. The following methods of professional learning in medicine are described in Step Three.

TYPE	METHOD
Academic activities	➤ Writing research papers ➤ Making presentations at conferences and seminars ➤ Refereeing journal articles ➤ Refereeing others' research bids ➤ Medico-legal activity ➤ Reading ➤ Writing and revising service and research protocols ➤ Acting as an external examiner ➤ Teaching
Meetings	➤ Clinical meetings: departmental and grand rounds ➤ Conferences ➤ Case review ➤ Post-mortems and the CPC ➤ Telephone and video conferences
Learning from colleagues	➤ Collaborative learning ➤ Consulting other professionals ➤ Joint ward rounds and clinics and professional conversations ➤ Library professionals ➤ Peer review ➤ Peer review: multiprofessional ➤ Peer tutoring ➤ Professional conversations ➤ Visits and travelling clubs ➤ Networking
Learning from practice	➤ Diaries ➤ Evidence-based practice ➤ Experiential learning ➤ Mistakes ➤ Opportunistic learning ➤ Portfolio-based learning ➤ Reflective learning

Technology-based learning and media	➤ Audio-visual ➤ Communication and information technologies ➤ Computer support systems ➤ Distance learning/blended learning ➤ Mass media and open sources ➤ Simulations ➤ Live interactive events ➤ Video review of performance ➤ Social media for learning
Management and quality processes	➤ Accreditation: hospital ➤ Audit ➤ Inspection visits ➤ Quality assessment schemes ➤ Revalidation
Specially arranged events	➤ Attachments and secondments ➤ Sabbaticals

Appendix 6: Methods of using the learning and showing its effects

Method	Main function			
	Use		To show effectiveness	
	Reinforcement of learning	Dissemination of learning*	For the organisation	For the doctor**
Accreditation/ certification of the individual				✔
Accreditation of services			✔	✔
Appraisal			✔	✔
Assessment of learning			✔	✔
Assessment results of trainees			✔	✔
Audit	✔	✔	✔	✔
Changes in person specification			✔	✔
Changing practice	✔	✔	✔	✔
Clinical effectiveness			✔	✔
CPD credit points				?
Collaborative assessment	✔	✔	✔	
Confidence levels				✔
Corporate image			✔	
Decreasing professional isolation				✔
'Don't know' factor			✔	✔

Educational culture			✔	
Educational records and log-books				?
Effects on the team			✔	✔
Enhancing practice	✔		✔	✔
Learning diaries	✔			✔
Learning portfolios	✔			✔
New services	✔	✔	✔	✔
Obsolete and inappropriate practice	✔	✔	✔	✔
Peer review of the medical team			✔	✔
Personal invigoration				✔
Protection from successful litigation			✔	✔
Recruitment of medical staff			✔	
Reduction in burnout and early retirement			✔	✔
Referrals to the doctor			✔	✔
Remunerative benefit				✔
Reporting back to colleagues	✔	✔	✔	✔
Reputation as a trainer			✔	✔
Research	✔	✔	✔	✔
Risk management	✔		✔	
Self-assessment	✔			✔
Time-efficient working			✔	✔
Video assessment	✔	✔		✔
Written reports	✔	✔		✔

*Dissemination of learning also implies effectiveness for the team or department.
**In most cases, this will also imply effectiveness for the institution in which the doctor works and so for patients.

Appendix 7: A personal development plan

Doctor:				Hospital/Practice:			
Department:				Specialty:			
GMC registration number:				Date:			
Plan for period from:				To:			
Proposals discussed with:				Date of appraisal/meeting:			
Proposed CPD activity	Date CPD activity was completed	How need was identified	How learning will be used and its effects determined?	Date follow-up was completed:	Full or partial CPD cycle completed?		Signed and dated by appraiser/ peer
1.					Full	Partial	
2.					Full	Partial	
3.					Full	Partial	
4.					Full	Partial	

References

1. Academy of Royal Medical Colleges. *Ten Principles for CPD*. London; 1999. Available at: www.aomrc.org.uk/ (accessed 24 August 2011).
2. General Medical Council (GMC) April 2004. *Guidance on Continuing Professional Development*. London; 2010. Available at: www.gmc-ukorg/education/pro development/pro development guidance.asp#principles (accessed 24 August 2011).
3. Lord Naren Patel. *Final Report of the Education and Training Regulation Policy Review: Recommendations and Options for the Future Regulation of Education and Training*. General Medical Council. London; 2010. Available at: www.gmc-uk.org/Recommendations and Options for the Future Regulation of Education and Training FINAL.pdf 31524263.pdf 34560875.pdf (accessed 24 August 2011).
4. McKay AJ. Revalidation: the catalyst for change in continuing professional development? *J Roy Coll Surg Edinb.* 2000; **45**(2): 71–3.
5. Bullock AD, Butterfield S, Belfield CR, *et al*. A role for clinical audit and peer review in the identification of continuing professional development needs for general dental practitioners: A discussion. *Brit Dent J.* 2000; **189**(8): 445–8.
6. General Medical Council. *Revalidation: The way ahead. Consultation Document*. London; 2010. www.gmc-uk.org/thewayahead (accessed 24 August 2011).
7. Davis N, Davis D, Bloch R. Continuing medical education: AMEE education guide no 35. *Med Teach.* 2008; **30**(7): 652–66.
8. Schostak J, Davis M, Hanson J, *et al*. The effectiveness of continuing professional development. A summary of findings. *Med Teach.* 2010; **32**: 586–92.
9. World Federation for Medical Education. *Continuing Professional Development of Medical Doctors 2003. WFME Global Standards for Quality Improvement*. University of Copenhagen; 2003. Available at: www3.sund.ku.dk/Activities/WFME%20CPD.pdf (accessed 24 August 2011).
10. Scally G, Donaldson LJ. Clinical governance and the drive for quality improvement in the new NHS in England. *BMJ.* 1998; **317**(7150): 61–5.
11. Hampton P. *Reducing administrative burdens: effective inspection and enforcement* 2005. HM Treasury, London; 2005. Available at: http://www.berr.gov.uk/files/file22988.pdf (accessed 24 August 2011).
12. Schostak J, Davis M, Hanson J, *et al*. *The Effectiveness of Continuing Professional Development. Final Report*. Academy of Medical Royal Colleges and The General Medical Council, London; 2010. Available at: www.gmc-uk.org/Effectiveness of CPD Final Report.pdf 34306281.pdf (accessed 24 August 2011).
13. General Medical Council. *Good Medical Practice*. London; 2006. Available at: www.gmc-uk.org/guidance/good medical practice/maintaining good medical practice up to date.asp (accessed 24 August 2011).
14. General Medical Council. *Proposals for Revalidation*. GMC, London; 2010. Available at: www.gmc-uk.org/4a Consultation on Revalidation.pdf 30284309.pdf (accessed 24 August 2011).

15. Pringle M. Revalidation: clearer and closer. *Brit J Gen Pract.* 2010; **60**(576): 475–6.

16. European Union of Medical Specialists. *Basel Declaration. UEMS Policy of Continuing Professional Development.* Brussels; 2001. Available at: www.uems.net/uploadedfiles/ 35.pdf (accessed 24 August 2011).

17. Nolan M, Owen R, Curran M, *et al.* Reconceptualising the outcomes of continuing professional development. *Int J Nurs Stud.* 2000; **37**: 457–67.

18. Grant J, Stanton F. *The Effectiveness of Continuing Professional Development. A Report for the Chief Medical Officer's Review of Continuing Professional Development in Practice.* Association for the Study of Medical Education. 2000. Available at: www.open.gov.uk/ doh/cmo/cmoh.htm (accessed 24 August 2011)

19. Davis DA, Thomson MA, Oxman AD, *et al.* Changing physician performance: A systematic review of the effect of continuing medical education strategies. *JAMA.* 1995; **274**: 700–5.

20. Grant J, Chambers E, Jackson G. *The Good CPD Guide. A Practical Guide to Managed CPD.* Sutton: Reed Healthcare Publishing; 1999.

21. Swedish Medical Association. *Better Continuing Professional Development – An Action Programme in Four Steps;* 2000. Available at: www.slf.se/Info-in-English/ (accessed 24 August 2011).

22. Amin Z. Theory and practice in continuing medical education. *Ann Acad Med Singap.* 2000; **29**(4): 4987–502.

23. Grant J. Learning needs assessment: assessing the need. *BMJ.* 2002; **324**(7330): 156–9.

24. Norman GR. The need for needs assessment in continuing medical education. *BMJ.* 2004; **328**: 999.

25. Grant J. The incapacitating effects of competence: a critique. *J Health Sci Educ.* 2000; **4**(3): 271–7.

26. Eve R. *PUNs and DENs. Discovering Learning Needs in General Practice.* Oxford: Radcliffe Medical Press; 2003.

27. Freeman R. *Mentoring in General Practice.* Oxford: Butterworth Heinemann; 1998.

28. Batstone G, Edwards M. Management of learning and professional development through clinical audit. In: White T, editor. *Textbook of Management for Doctors.* Edinburgh: Churchill Livingstone; 1996.

29. Davies H, Khera N, Stroobant J. Portfolios, appraisal, revalidation, and all that: a user's guide for consultants. *Arch Dis Child.* 2005; **90**: 165–70.

30. Regehr G, Eva K. Self-assessment, self-direction, and the self-regulating professional. *Clin Orthop Relat Res.* 2006; **449**: 34–8.

31. www.nbme.org/clinicians/benefits.html

32. Potter TB, Palmer RG. 360-degree assessment in a multidisciplinary team setting. *Rheumatol.* 2003; **42**(11): 1404–7.

33. Violato C, Lockyer J, Fidler H. Multisource feedback: a method of assessing surgical practice. *BMJ.* 2003; **326**: 546.

34. Pyatt RS, Moore DE, Caldwell SC. Improving outcomes through an innovative continuing medical education partnership. *JCEHP.* 1997; **17**: 239–44.

35. McClaran J, Snell L, Franco E. Type of clinical problem is a determinant of physicians' self-selected learning methods in their practice settings. *JCEHP.* 1998; **18**(2): 107–18.

36. Allery LA, Owen PA, Robling MR. Why general practitioners and consultants change their clinical practice. Critical incident survey. *BMJ.* 1997; **314**: 870–4.

37. Lave J, Wenger E. *Situated Learning. Legitimate peripheral participation.* Cambridge: University of Cambridge Press; 1991.

38. Macdonald MM. *Craft Knowledge in Medicine: An Interpretation of Teaching and Learning in Apprenticeship.* [Unpublished PhD Thesis]. Milton Keynes: Open University; 1998.

39. Page RL, Harrison BD. Interdepartmental peer review. *BMJ.* 1997; **314**(7083): 765–6.

40. Kolb DA, Rubin IM, Osland J. *Organizational Behavior: an experiential approach.* 5th ed. Englewood Cliffs, NJ: Prentice-Hall; 1991.

41. Knowles MS. Andragogy: an emerging technology for adult learning. In: Tight M, editor. *Adult Learning and Education.* London: Croom Helm; 1983.

42. Schön DA. *Educating the Reflective Practitioner.* 2nd ed. San Francisco, CA: Jossey-Bass; 1987.

43. Hewson MGAB. Reflection in clinical teaching: an analysis of reflection-on-action and its implications for staffing residents. *Med Teach.* 1991; **13**: 227–31.

44. Weerakoon PK, Fernando DN. Self-evaluation of skills as a method of assessing learning needs for continuing education. *Med Teach.* 1991; **13**: 103–6.

45. Dunn WR, Hamilton DD. Competence-based education and distance learning: a tandem for professional continuing education? *Stud High Educ.* 1985; **10**(2): 117–33.

46. Walton RT, Gierl C, Yudkin P, *et al.* Evaluation of computer support for prescribing (CAPSULE) using simulated cases. *BMJ.* 1997; **315**: 791–5.

47. Gordon J, Sanson-Fisher RW, Saunders NA. Identification of simulated patients by interns in a casualty setting. *Med Educ.* 1988; **22**: 533–8.

48. Bradley P, Bligh J. One year's experience with a clinical skills resource centre. *Med Educ.* 1999; **33**(2): 114–20.

49. Batstone G. Educational aspects of medical audit. *BMJ.* 1990; **301**: 326–8.

50. Davis DA, Thomson MA, Oxman AD, *et al.* Changing physician performance. A systematic review of the effect of continuing medical education strategies. *JAMA.* 1995; **274**(9): 700–5.

51. Irvine D. The performance of doctors 1. Professionalism and self-regulation in a changing world. *BMJ.* 1997; **314**(1): 540–2.

52. Griscti O, Jacono J. Effectiveness of continuing education programmes in nursing: literature review. *J Adv Nurs.* 2006; **55**(4): 449–56.

53. Marinopoulos SS, Dorman T, Ratanawongsa N, *et al.* Effectiveness of continuing medical education. *Evid Rep Tech Assess.* 2007; **149**: 1–69.

Index

360 degree assessment 34, 35, 78, 90, 138

Abernethy, RD 110
academic activities 22–3, 44–6
Academy of Medical Royal Colleges 8, 9, 117, 119
accreditation of hospitals 65
accreditation of services 74, 77
accreditation of the individual 34, 52, 74, 76–7, 116
action plans 55
acupuncture 67
adult learning theory 42, 57, 112
Advanced Trauma Life Support (ATLS) 76
adverse events 18, 26
Allery, L 109, 110, 123, 125
Al-Shehri, A 131
alternative medicine 67
American Board of Internal Medicine 35
Application Process Framework 140–1
appraisal
  appraisal record form template 157–9
  assessment of learning 78
  clinical governance 8
  enhancing practice 90
  how doctors identify learning needs 16
  identifying what to learn 13
  learning methods 39, 66
  needs assessment 20, 138
  planning how to learn 36, 37
  professional and regulatory environments 5
  reduction in burnout and early retirement 95
  using the learning 74, 77–8
apprenticeship learning 41, 54
Asian medical philosophy 67
ASPIRE study 83
assessment of learning 74, 78
assessment results of trainees 74, 78–9
ATLS (Advanced Trauma Life Support) 76
attachments 67
audio conferences 48–9

audio-visual modes of learning 59
audit
  learning methods 65
  needs assessment 18, 138
  problem of measurement 130
  professional and regulatory environments 5
  quality management 25–6
  using the learning 74, 79–80

Basel Declaration (EUMS) 9
Bath Information and Data Service (BIDS) 132
Beaudry, JS 125
behavioural event interview 58
Benett, Y 131
Bertram, DA 127
BIDS (Bath Information and Data Service) 132
blended learning 61–2
blind spots 17
blogs 64
Boud, DC 131
Branthwaite, A 110, 122
breast cancer 133
Bristol Royal Infirmary 111
British Cardiac Society 83
Brookfield, SD 112
Brooks-Bertram, PA 127
burnout 95–6
business plans 21

CAIPE *see* Centre for the Advancement of Interprofessional Education
cancer treatment 24, 133
cascade of benefits 95
case reviews 48
CDSR (Cochrane Database of Systematic Reviews) 55
Centre for the Advancement of Interprofessional Education (CAIPE) 116
certification of the individual 74, 76–7
Cervero, RM 112, 119, 120